FASTER CURES

———

FASTER CURES

Accelerating
the Future of Health

MICHAEL MILKEN

with

GEOFFREY EVANS MOORE

WILLIAM MORROW
An Imprint of HarperCollins*Publishers*

FIRST EDITION

Library of Congress Cataloging-in-Publication Data has been applied for.

ISBN 978-0-06-326021-4

23 24 25 26 27 LBC 5 4 3 2 1

To my grandchildren—Alice, Andie, Ari, Bailey, Hayden, Kylie, Maddie, Sloane, Spencer, and Stella—in the hope that our quest for faster cures will free you and everyone of your generation from having to face many of today's life-threatening diseases

Contents

Part IV: Priorities for the Future

Foreword

Winning the Battle

BY ANDREW VON ESCHENBACH, MD

––––––––––––

Less than seventy years ago, medicine as an art started to give way to medicine as a science. The inflection point was the discovery of DNA's structure. Before then, we could only observe the results of diseases, such as cancer, without having much in our arsenal to treat them effectively. The change occurred when medical scientists began to understand the mechanisms of disease at the genetic, molecular, and cellular level. A torrent of fundamental discoveries began to emerge from research laboratories.

Research, however, does not alleviate the suffering of patients. Research must be *translated* into clinical therapies before any of us can benefit. This involves grant applications, experimentation, publication, peer review, patenting, licensing, commercial investment, preclinical studies, clinical trials, regulatory review and approval, manufacturing, distribution, and more. By the early 1990s, discovery was rapidly outpacing this infrastructure for developing and delivering medical solutions. In one of the most fortuitous and profound coincidences of medical history, that's when Michael Milken assumed a leadership role—by transforming and accelerating the research and development process.

Mike was determined to improve the system, first for cancer and then for all life-threatening diseases. He wasn't alone in recognizing the problems—they were apparent to everyone in the field. What set him apart—what defined his genius—was the way he used a unique combination of energy, perceptiveness, and skill to create solutions. He advocated for and largely implemented new efficiencies and greater collaboration. That transformed the way many medical and scientific investigators did their work and exchanged data. No one in recent years has done more to advance the fight against serious disease.

The impact of organizations Mike launched—the Milken Family Foundation, the Milken Institute, CaP CURE, the Prostate Cancer Foundation, *FasterCures*, the Melanoma Research Alliance, and others—has been widely reported. Now he has wrapped them into the broader context of a lifetime's work. His narrative begins in childhood during the 1950s, moves on through his awakening to the tragic consequences of disease among family and friends, and then continues with his inspired efforts in medical research and public health that incorporated innovations he developed in finance.

Over the last thirty years, it has been my privilege to work in parallel with Mike on several of his initiatives to help accelerate a biomedical revolution. Thanks to that revolution, we now can not only detect and eliminate many diseases more successfully, but also prevent and control them. The tools we deploy are no longer limited to the life sciences—physical, computational, and materials sciences play a growing role.

Advances in medicine since the 1950s have been astounding: polio all but eliminated, heart disease cut in half, AIDS mostly controlled, cancer heading down, several hereditary defects corrected, COVID vaccines in record time. We should all be grateful to the dedicated researchers whose work has helped give us extra decades to enjoy life. That, says Mike Milken, is only the beginning. Exponential progress lies ahead as new discoveries arrive with breathtaking speed. Some therapies now entering the clinic would have been considered science fiction less than a decade ago. As a result, millions of patients are living longer.

Mike's personal journey, as told in this memoir, is an enlightening reflection on the path of progress. It is even more valuable as a road map to a future in which patients' hopes become reality.

Following three decades as an oncologist, surgeon, and medical executive, Dr. Andrew C. von Eschenbach was named director of the National Cancer Institute in 2001. From 2006 to 2009, he served as commissioner of the United States Food and Drug Administration. He is currently president of Samaritan Health Initiatives and an adjunct professor at the University of Texas MD Anderson Cancer Center.

Introduction

The Rivers of a Life

Three rivers converge near downtown Pittsburgh. The Allegheny rises from a spring on Cobb Hill in Potter County, Pennsylvania. It widens and deepens when joined by many tributaries as it races southwest to unite with the Monongahela. Their confluence becomes a third major river—the Ohio—and continues for another thousand miles through the heart of America. Hundreds of smaller streams add volume.

Sometimes my life seems like a river with three main tributaries of interest—science, education, and access to capital. These commingled with personal values—commitment to family and community— instilled by my parents. Over time, science focused increasingly on medical research and public health; education on student achievement and teacher development; business on job creation and the democratization of finance. Thousands of friends and associates contributed to the mix, each a stream that influenced and enlarged the whole.

This book invites you to join me on a personal journey highlighting stories of challenges and triumphs in medical science. Some of our initiatives in education and finance are also part of the narrative because they help define me. But this is not an autobiography. I intend to write a future volume on education—including development of the Milken Center for Advancing the American Dream and such programs as the Milken Educator Awards, the Milken Scholars, and the International Finance Corporation–Milken Institute Capital Markets Program.

My future plans also include a third book covering my years on Wall Street, beginning in 1969, which have been chronicled extensively, but not accurately. Those years ended with a prosecution that manufactured a false profile of me—it was the antithesis of how I lived my life and who I am. The process even held members of my family hostage. Under intense public scrutiny that affected my loved ones, I decided not to drag it out through years of fighting in court as others who prevailed chose to do. Although I was incarcerated for twenty-two months, my lifelong dedication to the democratization of capital was undiminished. That mission simply shifted to the non-profit arena with the launch of the Milken Institute. I look forward to writing about this. As the English philosopher Francis Bacon said, "Truth is the daughter of time, not of authority."

WHAT THIS BOOK IS ABOUT

The stories in the following chapters tell of important events in my life. The early innovations in finance turned out to be a template for much of what we've accomplished in the search for faster cures.* That

---

* "No man is an island," wrote John Donne. If we achieve anything, it is only with the help of others. This presents a dilemma for an author who writes about his own experiences

search includes our programs to accelerate the work of medical pioneers whose achievements have changed the course of history.

I'll also touch briefly on other issues involved in my financial work: what I saw that others missed in the capacity of certain innovations to create jobs. Why, despite initial resistance to those innovations, they became the foundation for much of the world's financial markets. When we provided financing for such key industries as cable, cellular phones, energy, healthcare, housing, media, and telecommunications, the goal was more than wealth creation. Everyone who worked with me understood that no matter what level of success we achieved, we all wanted meaningful lives for our children; and they wouldn't have that unless *all* children in society had an opportunity. That understanding is the basis of the American dream. It provides the motivation for building our Center for Advancing the American Dream.

Here I've written about matters of health including the emotional devastation of my father's fatal illness and my children's medical issues. How my life (and the life of my wife, Lori) was turned upside down when we thought our first son might die and when our daughter was born very small and fragile. How we bonded with parents everywhere who can never rest when faced with such unpredictable threats as childhood epilepsy, life-threatening allergies, or type 1 diabetes.

One of my goals is to provide you with useful information and a realistic perspective because you and your family, like all families, have had to deal with life-threatening issues (or will someday). Financial resources can help, but they do little to prepare people for the emotional burden of disease. I would have traded all my financial

---

without resorting to constant use of the first person singular. It would be unfair to omit the contributions of others when I was often one of many responsible for a project's success. Yet frequent use of compound subjects like "my colleagues and I" becomes tedious. Instead, the stories within often begin sentences with "we" as shorthand for the hundreds of managers and professionals who have worked with me over the years. Their dedication to speeding the search for cures has earned my lasting respect and admiration.

success if it could have saved my father's life, brought back other relatives and friends stricken in their prime, or cleared an easier path for my children. Perhaps my experiences can lighten some of the burden for others.

You'll read about our meetings with health leaders, industry CEOs, government officials, and others as we developed new strategies and figured out what could work. You'll see why we rejected the advice of the American Cancer Society, which initially thought our 1998 March on Washington would "fragment the movement." And you'll understand why, a dozen years later, we used a totally different strategy to convene the leaders of bioscience in an innovation retreat and then—a year after that—to reenergize the nation's commitment in what we called the Celebration of Science.

There's nothing wrong with writing checks to support good causes. We've done it extensively. But such charitable giving is not enough to change the underlying research process. Instead, we set out to build a more effective and efficient research infrastructure; to create a model that others could use in pursuit of faster solutions for all life-threatening diseases.

We began by recruiting top scientists and physicians to careers in medical research and public health, making it easier and more worthwhile for them to communicate with each other, and removing bureaucratic roadblocks that impeded their efforts. Our funding jump-started the process so that others, including government and industry, would follow our lead. In the search for faster cures that save lives, we worked to make the scientific, translational, and clinical processes more fulfilling and productive pursuits.

The message to other health advocates, foundations, and disease-specific organizations was inclusive. We invited them to join our efforts toward substantially increasing funding for every type of medical research. They had a front-row seat at our planning meetings for events like the March on Washington, the Celebration of

Science, our Future of Health Summits, and relevant panels at the annual Milken Institute Global Conferences. We didn't ask these other groups to help fund events, but always sought their input. The idea was that by sharing our thinking on how to improve the research process, we would all benefit.

In 1998, we told these organizations that everyone stood to gain if Congress doubled the National Institutes of Health budget, which was an important goal of that summer's March on Washington. The March itself focused on cancer, not because noncancerous diseases were less worthy of support, but because cancer would draw the greatest attention on Capitol Hill. It was—and remains—a condition that touches nearly every family, including the families of senators, representatives, and their staffs. But every disease-specific group, we assured them, would be part of our campaign.

WHY HEALTH AND MEDICAL RESEARCH?

The focus on health and medical research is important because:

- Health affects everyone on the planet. With improved medical outcomes, we will be able to pass along more of our knowledge, wisdom, and life experiences to future generations. Effective health interventions improve the *quality* of life in addition to its length.

- Medical research has intersected with every stage of my life from childhood awareness of polio in the 1950s through our recent efforts to accelerate cures for a wide range of diseases.

- We've all learned crucial public health lessons from the COVID-19 pandemic. It has tested everything we thought we knew about treating disease and has shown the inestimable value of long-term research. Decades of previous investments underlay the astonishingly rapid development of vaccines and therapies.

+ The future of bioscience is incredibly promising. We can look forward to great progress in such areas as cancer, the brain, the immune system, and infectious diseases. Scientists working on multi-cancer early detection have developed technologies that will save countless lives. Others are beginning to understand the fundamental mechanisms of aging. It's a magnificent opportunity: For the first time in history, we can realistically aspire to eliminate much of the burden of serious disease. It won't be easy.

One goal of this book is to share what has driven me for five decades . . . and what I've learned from that work. The original "blueprint" for my life—to borrow a phrase from a 1967 Martin Luther King Jr. speech—was to become a scientist or an astronaut. Then a dramatic 1965 encounter altered it. The blueprint changed again in the 1970s when a series of family medical issues refocused my goals. My own terminal cancer diagnosis in 1993 led to yet another change in my approach to medical research. On reflection, I have a better understanding of why my lifelong quest to speed the pace of discovery has been so central to who I am. My own process of self-discovery led me to the conclusion that medicine can now offer people controls and cures for life-threatening diseases within their own lifetimes. In other words, we can discover cures faster than the historical trend suggests.

Remember that science as we know it, especially medicine, has evolved only over the past two centuries and the *rate* of change is accelerating. As recently as the nineteenth century, people suffered through gruesome surgeries without anesthesia, childbirth without antiseptic procedures, and all manner of intractable infections. Fortunately, medicine has advanced from that dark past to the prospect of a bright future that will transform society in the years ahead.

A theme woven throughout these pages is the triumph of science over conventional wisdom and fear. At the height of the 1950s polio epidemic, economists predicted that the twentieth century would end with America spending $100 billion a year on "iron lung hotels." Diagnosed with lung cancer in 1964, the actor John Wayne told the world he had "the big C" and everyone assumed his death was imminent. (He lived another fifteen years and made more than twenty additional movies.) In the 1980s, one analysis estimated that, by the year 2000, AIDS patients would fill half of all hospital beds. In 2020, the COVID pandemic instilled such fear that officials in California speculated about two million future deaths in that state alone.

Science met these challenges in the form of the Salk and Sabin polio vaccines, public health campaigns, statins, antiretroviral therapy cocktails, advanced nutrition, genome sequencing, immunotherapies, monoclonal antibodies, mRNA vaccines, noninvasive surgeries, powerful new diagnostic scans, artificial intelligence, and CRISPR gene editing.

My professional journey, beginning in the 1960s, intersected with many of these advances. My *personal* journey, however, began a decade earlier in a typical mid-century American family. It proceeded through childhood adventures; the influence of my father's early struggles; the collegiate free-speech movement; an awakening to the roots of social disparities; the challenges of a young parent; and success in my financial career.

The middle sections of this book describe a major health crisis and how it accelerated my work on a broad campaign to strengthen the impact of medical research and public health. (*Fortune* magazine said it "changed medicine.") The later chapters look at emerging technologies, the lessons of COVID-19, and prospects for a healthier future. I conclude with some thoughts on meaningful lives.

THE GREATEST ACHIEVEMENT

The idea for this volume began with a look back on five decades of interaction with thousands of patients and professionals in medicine, science, and public health. To understand the importance of their efforts, consider this question: **What is the greatest achievement in the history of civilization?** Some would argue it's the invention of the wheel, the origination of agriculture, or the evolution of communication from cave drawings to the printing press to the internet. Others might cite such concepts as the development of trade, the rule of law, and democracy.

These are epochal accomplishments. But in my opinion, the greatest achievement is the twentieth and twenty-first centuries' worldwide extension of life spans and improvements in quality of life. You can understand just how remarkable this is by comparing the rapid progress in the last century to the slow advance of longevity over four million years since the appearance of the first prehuman hominids. Today, it's not unusual to have great-grandchildren.

Our earliest ancestors survived for about twenty years. By 1900, people throughout the world lived an average of only thirty-one years, although it was forty-seven in the United States. Of course, that average was reduced by the prevalence of infant mortality, especially in poverty-stricken developing nations. Still, it's surprising that in the entire development of our species up until 1900, the *average* increased only eleven years.

One hundred years later—the blink of an eye in evolutionary terms—life spans on earth had more than doubled to sixty-seven. Today they're about seventy-four worldwide. Some countries have achieved averages as high as eighty-five. In Monaco, it's almost ninety. We reached these milestones mostly by preventing and cur-

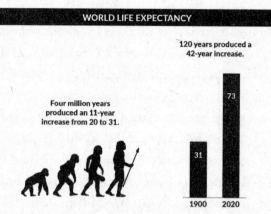

WORLD LIFE EXPECTANCY

120 years produced a
42-year increase.

Four million years
produced an 11-year
increase from 20 to 31.

73

31

1900   2020

ing more than a dozen infectious diseases that plagued humans for millennia.

As recently as 1900, one out of every five newborns in America died before celebrating a fifth birthday. The leading causes of death were pneumonia, tuberculosis, and enteritis with diarrhea—all infectious. Thanks largely to progress in sanitation and the development of vaccines and antibiotics, those diseases are now far less common. Today, at least four of every five people live into their sixties and death comes most often from cardiovascular disease and cancer. Happily, the burden of heart conditions and many types of cancer has fallen sharply.

There's also a remarkable economic benefit. In real, inflation-adjusted terms, the per capita productivity of advanced economies is eight times that of the nineteenth-century average. **And half of all economic growth over the past two hundred years is directly linked to progress in medical research and public health.**[*]

That's a key reason for the focus of this first book. Some financial market prognosticators tend to overlook health's economic sig-

---

* The late British economic historian Angus Maddison calculated these facts in his monumental work, *The World Economy: A Millennial Perspective* (OECD, 2001).

nificance by citing recent "disruptive" technologies as the basis for growth. Of course it's true that advances in communications, energy, and mobility supported much economic expansion since 1900. That growth would have been greatly diminished, however, if not for the improved health and longevity of the population.

Unfortunately, the benefits of medical and public health advances are not evenly distributed around the world. Those of us in the wealthier nations live years, often decades, longer than the average African, Latin American, or South Asian. And serious health inequities persist in the developed world. The Milken Institute's programs to address both of these disparities have made some headway. In February 2020, before the COVID-19 pandemic fully emerged as a massive global crisis, we had just spent ten days in the Middle East and Africa. We went there to work on advancing economic development and public health.

The long flight back from Johannesburg, South Africa, to Los Angeles gave me time to outline some of the ways the Institute and our related medical organizations could contribute to solutions for what was starting to look like a major pandemic. How, I asked, might our experiences in medical science and public health be deployed? One idea was to combine everything I'd learned over the previous five decades with the insights of others who were leading the COVID-19 battle. The result is a series of podcasts that frame the issues, point to solutions, and outline strategies. (These podcasts and transcripts are at www.fastercuresbook.com.)

MY PERSONAL JOURNEY

This book is a narrative of *hope*. Not just the hope of longer lives, but also healthier, more meaningful lives for people everywhere. The concluding chapter brings the narrative full circle by focusing on a single recent day that encompassed the three rivers of my life as reflected in the achievements of several extraordinary people.

The poet William Wordsworth famously wrote, "The child is father of the man." So this personal journey begins in childhood, a time when my innate curiosity was nurtured. It helps explain the path that took me to the frontiers of medical science . . . and beyond.

PART I

Preparing for Today's Challenges

Setting the Stage

———

"Optimistic" seems the best way to describe the America I knew in the 1950s. Having confronted the Great Depression and World War II, my mom and dad, like many young parents, felt their children would inherit a better world.

When I was born in 1946—one of the first baby boomers—we lived in an apartment near downtown LA. Two years later, we moved to a larger apartment when my brother, Lowell, was born. Then, in 1952, our family joined thousands of other Los Angeles households moving "over the hill" to a house in the more affordable San Fernando Valley. We settled in the middle-class community of Encino.

Lowell and I shared a bedroom in our house on Densmore Avenue. Although only about 1,300 square feet, it was a nurturing home for our close family. My parents liked to host monthly dinner-and-bridge parties for a group of their friends. Eight couples sat at four card tables in our combined living-dining room.

The game of bridge requires knowledge, intuition, and common sense to figure out the cards in other people's hands. I had learned how to play and loved the game because it combined quantitative knowledge (counting the cards) and qualitative assessment of what different players are likely to do (how they bid and play their hands). Of course, I wasn't part of this competition, but I had a different competition in my mind one autumn Saturday night in 1954 when I was eight. After preparing all week, my excitement grew as the weekend approached. I planned to talk to these adults about facts and trends from my favorite book, the *World Almanac and Book of Facts*. Because the rules of bridge decree that one of the four players at each table bows out of the game at a certain point in each hand, there was always someone to engage on my own. Sometimes I'd just quiz that player about a fact gleaned from my reading. But my goal wasn't to stump the adult; it was to learn about how the world worked (and how it was changing)—to learn not just what happened, but *why* things happened.

The guests arrived after Lowell's bedtime, but as the older boy, I was allowed to stay up later. This would be my only chance for another month. Of course, I could ask them about things like the names of past presidents, the year women got the vote, or the distance to the nearest star. Like most kids who read science fiction comics, I knew the speed of light and plenty of other science facts. But that would just be showing off. Better to learn by seeing the world through other people's eyes. These adults could teach me things beyond schoolwork; things I could later discuss with Mom and Dad at the dinner table.

From the time I could read, facts had fascinated me. I couldn't wait until the mail carrier delivered the almanac once a year. Many nights, I'd read it with a flashlight under the covers.

Then my parents bought an entire encyclopedia set. It had thousands, *tens* of thousands of facts jammed into two dozen volumes I could pick up and savor!

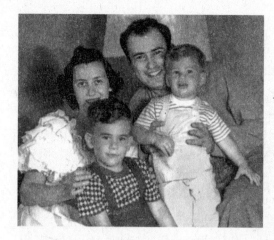

At age 4, with my parents and younger brother Lowell.

However, the encyclopedia had a major drawback: it quickly went out of date. The advantage of the almanac was that it showed how the world was *changing* year to year. I learned all the state capitals, the deepest lakes, the highest mountains. Interesting facts, but unchanging. I was more interested in how the world was changing year to year. The populations of some countries grew faster than others; America produced more or fewer cars in certain years; the stock market rose and fell. I wanted to know what was behind these changes.

Later, in junior high school math, I would learn that the first derivative of any equation is the amount it changes over time; and the second derivative is the change in the *rate* of change. Intuitively, this is what my eight-year-old mind was grasping as I compared facts from different years.

It would be another fifteen years before I concluded that "The Best Investor Is a Social Scientist," the title of my first speech on Wall Street. Yet looking back, it's clear that my early childhood curiosity—that hunger for learning—was where it started. I wanted to assimilate diverse facts into useful social theories.

Still, sometimes I couldn't resist producing a number or date so obscure it would startle the adults.

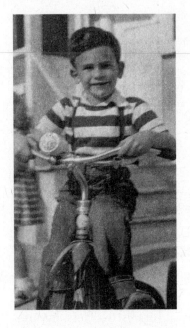

On my way (age 5).

One of the bridge players considered himself a real expert on baseball. He talked about it all the time. This Saturday night, he mentioned an amazing over-the-shoulder catch that the great Willie Mays had made a few days earlier in Game One of the 1954 World Series at New York's Polo Grounds. It remains one of the most famous defensive plays in baseball history. Aha! An opening for a question: Can anyone tell me how far deepest center field is from home plate at the Polo Grounds? What a disappointment that no one knew it was 483 feet.

At dinner before the bridge game that night, the adults discussed the recent Supreme Court decision in *Brown v. Board of Education* declaring racial segregation in schools to be unconstitutional. Even though they had strong opinions about the case, no one came close to having the correct answer when I asked a related question based on a statistic I had read: What percent of the US population were non-white minorities?* Almost everyone guessed about twenty percent—nearly double the actual figure of 10.5 percent. Nobody, I concluded, knows everything. It was the first, but not the last, time

---

* Even as late as 1960, 75 percent of US immigrants came from Europe. Today, only 9 percent are from Europe while about 83 percent are from Latin America or Asia. Some 38 percent of today's total US population is non-white.

I had this feeling. Later in life, I learned that most people's knowledge of "facts" was usually based on what someone else had told them, not on firsthand experience or research.

Why didn't these wise people know the answers? They were intelligent adults and weren't shy about expressing their views on events they'd heard about in the news. Yet even with all the years they'd had to learn, they didn't know much of the information that was so easy to look up. It seemed illogical.

As I would eventually come to understand, many things that seem logical are not always true. It seems logical that financial markets adjust interest rates in exact proportion to risk; that stress causes ulcers; that bed rest should be prescribed for heart-attack survivors; or that red meat is the best source of dietary protein. All seem logical. All are wrong.

THE JOY OF NUMBERS

Interpreting facts was always part of my family's nightly dinner table conversation. Not facts for their own sake, but information that helped make sense of the world. We'd discuss the latest TV shows, or global events, or how postwar economic expansion and the baby boom were affecting my father's business clients. As an accountant and a lawyer, he saw their changing fortunes up close. He gave my brother Lowell and me an early understanding of the risks entrepreneurs took every day. He'd quiz me about what I'd learned in class and show genuine interest in my elementary school lessons.

As early as kindergarten, I liked numbers and was always proud to demonstrate my math skills. Just as some people who have a feel for music become composers, I had a feel for math and knew I wanted a career that included it—probably as a scientist. Handheld calculators hadn't yet been invented, but arithmetic and algebra were easy to do in my head.

Numbers seemed thrilling and became my passion. No wonder I dreamed of space travel. Alpha Centauri, the nearest star, is twenty-five *trillion* miles from Earth.

Let's see, I thought, that would be about 300,000 times the distance from Earth to the sun!

At the speed of light, it's 4.367 years away. To me, these were important facts because if something happened to the Earth or the sun, humans would have to find a home somewhere else in the universe.*

One of my happiest family outings was when my parents took me to the Griffith Observatory, not far from our home. If you visited at the right time, you could play explorer, like Columbus or Magellan. We'd sit under the planetarium dome and when they turned out the lights, stars would appear on the ceiling. The challenge was to navigate an imaginary boat as the stars moved so you ended up at the right destination. It was one more experience that strengthened my desire to pursue science.

Some of my favorite comic books portrayed brave interstellar travelers. My collection featured plenty of fantasy heroes from DC and Marvel: Superman, Batman, the Green Lantern and the Space Ranger. I was fascinated by their quest for something greater than mere mortals could achieve. A favorite childhood movie was *Forbidden Planet*, released in 1956, which I rank among the all-time greats of science fiction. Its message: Technology without humanity or compassion is useless. That struck a chord with me as a kid . . . and it still does.

---

* My childhood fantasy came full circle at the 2016 Milken Institute Global Conference, when the entrepreneur, physicist and technology investor Yuri Milner presented Breakthrough Starshot, a plan to develop a "light sail" craft able to make the journey to Alpha Centauri at one-fifth the speed of light.

SUMMER CAMP

Los Angeles has always been a diverse city—dozens of different languages are spoken in the homes of LA public school students. Our Encino neighborhood, which included families from different socioeconomic levels, had a real sense of community. Neighbors looked out for each other and their children. When I was ten years old, my mother didn't think twice about letting me take off on my bicycle. I rode my bike the six blocks to Hesby Street Elementary School as well as to visit friends, play in Little League games, and collect dimes and quarters from neighbors as a student volunteer for the local Community Chest fundraising drive. (Today, it's called the United Way.)

My friends and I had a great time just being kids. But our parents felt we needed more structure. There were few summer day camps for kids in the area and none in our neighborhood. In 1953, several neighbors decided to start their own camp. They called it Vista Stars. My lifelong friend Richard Sandler (now executive vice president of the Milken Family Foundation), was only five years old; at the time, I was seven, one of the "older kids." The Sandlers had a two-acre back lot that became Vista Stars headquarters.

They hired Ray O'Conner to be the camp counselor. Ray was a former UCLA baseball star who later played professionally for three years until injuries ended that career. Determined to toughen us up and teach us a few things about life, he put us to work with hoes and rakes to create a baseball field. It was hard, sweaty work for two weeks, but Ray's response to any complaint was "Don't be a baby!" When the field was complete, we were proud of the result.

Even then, a game like baseball got me thinking mathematically. *How many feet around all four bases? What is the speed of a fastball? Is the arc of a fly ball a parabola? What was Ted Williams's batting average?* There was data everywhere!

We toughened up over the years in summer camp and learned about determination. If one of us fell down and scraped a knee, Ray would bark, "Shake it off and get back in the game." During one practice a few years later, Richard tripped and landed on his arm while chasing a fly ball. Afraid to show how much it hurt, he finished the afternoon in pain. Only when his mother took him to a doctor did he learn that he had broken his wrist.

Later, when I played on the neighborhood Little League team, I was one of the best hitters . . . and one of the worst fielders. (Unfortunately, the designated hitter rule didn't exist yet.) So I got to see a lot of right field, where I could do the least harm. Win or lose, though, I always enjoyed the opportunity to compete. Whenever things got tough later in life, a voice in the back of my head said, "Shake it off and get back in the game."

BASEBALL AND BOLSHEVIKS

The nostalgic view of the 1950s is one of a simpler time. Television was pretty much limited to CBS, NBC, or ABC.* Most people drove a Chevy, Ford, or Plymouth and there were only a few flavors of ice cream. If that seems constraining, consider the choices in phone companies: There was no choice. If you wanted a telephone, you got it

---

* The nearly unlimited entertainment and communications options we enjoy today—hundreds of television channels, immediate and low-cost conferencing and messaging to anyone anywhere in the world, high-definition on-demand movies at our fingertips—all were birthed in the Great Communications Revolution of the 1970s, '80s, and '90s. It was my honor to team up with many of the remarkable entrepreneurs who led this revolution. Their stories will be among those featured at the Milken Center for Advancing the American Dream.

from Ma Bell (and the instrument was black, thank you very much).*
To send a package across the country, you drove to the train station
and filled out forms in triplicate at the Railway Express Agency. No
one I knew had ever made an international phone call, maybe because it cost about twelve dollars a minute at a time when the average
take-home pay was less than a hundred dollars a week.

Major League Baseball was something played east of the Missis-
sippi. As far as New York sports writers were concerned, we might
as well have been living on the moon. But in the fall of 1957, Los Angeles was abuzz with talk of the Brooklyn Dodgers, whose pending
arrival for the following season confirmed that Los Angeles really
was a big-league city.

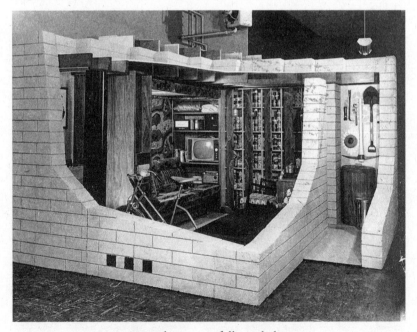

1950s basement fallout shelter.

---

* I thought back to this when, in the early 1980s, I financed MCI's Bill McGowan and his
vision of a future that wouldn't be dominated by one telephone company.

It was a good time and place to be a kid despite the lack of protection by seat belts, childproof bottle caps, and bicycle helmets. According to advertisements in *Life* and *Look* magazines, even smoking was benign. One ad proclaimed, "More doctors smoke Camels than any other cigarette!"

Much public concern centered on the threat of communism—an ominous word often capitalized in newspaper stories of the day—especially the brand practiced by the Russians, who now possessed "the bomb." After the Soviet Union tested a hydrogen weapon in 1953, we began to hear of neighbors building fallout shelters to protect against airborne radioactive matter. So imminent was the perceived danger that we dutifully practiced duck-and-cover drills in school.

At one school assembly, the flickering movie-screen image of Bert, a goofy-looking turtle, showed us how it was done. He hid under his shell while a chorus sang a catchy jingle about ducking under our desks.

But I was skeptical that ducking and covering would do any good when atomic weapons started flying. I made that clear to our sixth-

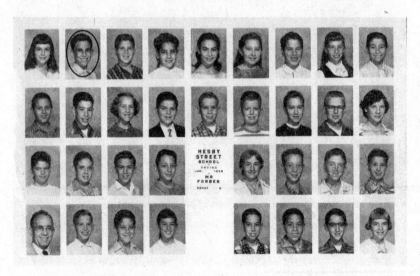

Sixth grade with one of my favorite teachers, Mr. Forbes.

grade teacher, Mr. Forbes. A patient man, he became annoyed when I constantly challenged the logic of crouching under our desks as protection from a bomb falling on Hesby Street School. One day, I spoke up so loudly that everyone's eyes turned toward me. Peering over his glasses, Mr. Forbes said we'd talk about it after school. Following some private negotiating, we reached an agreement: I promised not to disrupt the class and Mr. Forbes said he wouldn't try to convince me I'd be safe under my desk.

Hesby Street had wonderful teachers—especially Mr. Sutton and Mrs. Friedman. I loved the sights, the sounds, the smells of the school. The formal portraits of thirty-four US presidents stared down from above the blackboards; our ancient desks still had inkwells; the bell of the Good Humor truck outside the window made us salivate like Pavlov's dogs; chalk dust floated in the morning sun; and the aroma of macaroni and cheese announced the lunch menu long before we reached the cafeteria.

While math and science had a special appeal to me, I also loved the big, colorful maps with exotic names like Belgian Congo. I devoured the facts, committing to memory the capitals, rivers, and mountain ranges. But I also analyzed *relative* information.

In one class, we were paired off to play "the map game." Two at a time, we'd stand with our backs to the wall. When the teacher called out the name of a city or country, we'd whirl around to see which of us could find it first. It was a fun game, but it also made me think about why some geographically small nations like England were bigger industrial powers than others with more land area. Why was the population of India so much greater than Australia's even though its land mass was smaller? What was happening *within* countries? What made some European nations more successful than others in recovering from the devastation of World War II?

Dominating the world map was a huge red blob labeled "Union of Soviet Socialist Republics." It stretched across eleven time zones and dwarfed the United States. It was the biggest country in the world and many newspapers would have us believe it was overflowing with atom bombs. But at least those bombs were thousands of miles and a Pacific Ocean away from Encino. And I was reassured that Dwight Eisenhower, the famous wartime general, was in the White House.

California, like the rest of the country, seemed a safe place.

SPUTNIK: THE WAKE-UP CALL FROM SPACE

In 1957, none of us doubted that Americans were the best at everything. Our factories were humming, the US. military was powerful, our technology and consumer goods were the envy of every nation. US-based scientists had been awarded the most Nobel Prizes, by far. With less than 6 percent of the world's population, the US produced nearly 40 percent of global economic output, up from less than 2 percent early in the nineteenth century. Everywhere in the world, people watched American movies and listened to our music. We boasted of more telephones, television sets, cars, bathtubs, and refrigerators than any place on earth. Students came from every country to study at our great universities. Not since ancient Rome had any nation dominated so many aspects of life on the planet.

But on the morning of Friday, October 4, 1957, an electronic signal from 560 miles above Earth told the world that the Soviets had beaten America into space. "Reds Launch Artificial Moon" was a typical headline. The scary thing about the satellite, which Russians called "Sputnik," wasn't the 184-pound aluminum sphere that did little more than beep at us. The real threat was the Soviet R-7 intercontinental missile that blasted it up there only two months after the first successful test firing. Within days of Sputnik, Soviet leader Nikita Khrushchev boasted that his nation would begin turning out nuclear-tipped missiles "like sausages." America suddenly realized that its most powerful enemy now had the capacity to hurl lethal weapons across the oceans.

Hesby Street School now didn't seem like such a safe place after all.

It was frightening, but it obscured important facts. At the time of Sputnik, the USSR's gross domestic product was no larger than the economies of a few small US states like Massachusetts and Maryland. It was interesting for me to see the different ways people reacted to the news. Some were intrigued by the scientific achievement; but many, including a number of my sixth-grade classmates, were terrified. A book by Paul Dickson, *Sputnik: The Shock of the Century* (Walker Books, 2007), said it created more national anxiety than any event since Pearl Harbor.

By shocking America's complacent educational and technology infrastructures, Sputnik triggered immense US reforms that helped put Americans on the moon a dozen years later. It also accelerated development of revolutionary new technologies.

With the benefit of hindsight, we know that Moscow's moment of apparent triumph turned out to be the beginning of the end for the Soviet communist system. The very event that was intended to demonstrate Soviet superiority became our wake-up call. And wake up we did. President Eisenhower soon signed the National Defense Education Act. NDEA stimulated studies in science, mathematics and Slavic languages with generous aid to public and private education. Its funding paid for a sweeping curriculum overhaul, language labs, new math courses, scientific fellowships, and increased student loans. The act injected billions of dollars into US high schools and colleges during the 1960s. So intent was America on meeting the Soviet challenge that even physical fitness courses came to be seen as a means to defeat the Russians. All this stimulated student interest in scientific careers—it was something "cool" they could aspire to.

Congress soon established DARPA—the Defense Advanced Research Projects Agency—and NASA—the National Aeronautics and Space Administration.* Both organizations were created to assure that America would never again fall behind in scientific and military leadership. NASA folded together and oversaw space projects that had been under the control of the Naval Research Laboratory, the army, and the air force. We were in the scientific equivalent of wartime. The following decades would have been very different if we hadn't heeded the call and bent the arc of history. As President Kennedy famously declared a few years later, "We shall pay any price, bear any burden, meet any hardship . . . to assure the survival and success of liberty."

And amid all this government action, ordinary citizens took up the banner, too. I may have been only eleven when Sputnik was launched, but that didn't stop me from writing a letter to President Eisenhower offering my services in America's future space program. After all, my letter noted, I could quickly multiply up to four digits in my head, I'd never missed a math or science problem, and I'd learned all about space from my visits to Griffith Observatory.

I was disappointed when the White House didn't reply. But I wasn't alone in my enthusiasm. Science *itself* was practically a hero to kids back then, particularly the applied technology type that dealt with exciting fields like rocketry. (I was fascinated by such problems as the required velocity to send a rocket into orbit.) It seemed that inventions to solve every problem were just around the corner.

It was a golden age for anyone with talent who wanted to make contraptions that go fast. Some kids started designing experiments

---

* Little did I know then that decades later the Milken Institute and our medical foundations would work with both agencies on projects related to medical science; or that I'd find myself on a Moscow stage debating the Russian leader Vladimir Putin. (This was long before he directed the Russian invasions of Crimea and Ukraine. At the time, US-Russia relations were still relatively cordial.) During a discussion of Sputnik, I remember that President Putin corrected my pronunciation from *Spuht-nick* to what sounded like *Schpoot-neek* [Простейший Спутник]. He continued to insist that Sputnik proved the superiority of what was then the Soviet system.

with bicycle spokes, matchstick tips, and tin cans—then graduated to crystal radios, Tesla coils, vacuum pumps, and backyard miniature rockets. Most of them grew up with all their fingers and toes intact.

Some of us were concerned the Russians might possess death rays like the ones in our comic books. (Actually, it wasn't too different from what the Pentagon feared.) But mostly we were excited about the future of science, and our dreams grew bigger every day. One of the great strengths of science is its power to make us dream. Some kids may have planned to become firefighters or veterinarians; my dream was to travel in space.

Throughout all this, I was doing research, accumulating more information, not realizing that data would be central to my later parallel careers in finance and medical research. It was training for a lifetime of applying data to the solution of problems.

TWO

Shaping My Beliefs:
Family and Community

———————

My dad was an active man. He loved to dance, enjoyed coaching our Little League baseball team, and often joined in other sports. One day when I was about eight or nine, he was throwing a football around with my friends and me. One kid blurted out, "Hey, what's wrong with your father's leg? He has a limp." Really? I'd never noticed. But sure enough, there was this hitch in his gait.

After dinner that night, we talked about it.

Sitting in the living room, I asked, "Dad, how come you limp?" He explained that he'd contracted polio as an infant, leaving him with a leg that was not fully developed. (Thinking about it later, I realized that he always wore long pants. Despite our mild California weather, I'd never seen him in shorts.) With this revelation, he must have determined that I was old enough to process even more disturbing information because he opened up about other details of his life. It was quite a story, and difficult for him to tell.

I already knew that times had been tough during the Great Depression, and that I'd never met my paternal grandparents. When Dad was three years old, his mother died during childbirth. The baby, who would have been his brother, also died. Several years later, his father perished in an auto accident and Dad was sent to live in a home for orphaned boys. Added to all that was the realization that entire branches of our extended family had perished in the Holocaust. Those emotional traumas instilled in him a powerful appreciation for a close and loving family, a constant theme of his dinner table conversation.

I was devastated by all this information. Up until that point, I hadn't thought much about polio. My parents had often warned me not to swim in neighbors' pools or drink from water fountains. They were trying to protect me and I guess I hadn't appreciated their efforts. The disease had been an abstraction to me, something that happened to other people.

Now that I found out my own father was a victim, I became obsessed with studying polio—how you got it, who was affected, when it became an epidemic, what it did to the body, how a vaccine was developed . . . everything. When my mother took me to our pediatrician, I bombarded him with questions about polio. That was the first time I was doing research on a disease.

That one evening talking with Dad had a profound effect on the rest of my life. It made me realize just how lucky I was to live in an era when vaccines provide protection against a long list of diseases that used to be debilitating or fatal; and it motivated me to work toward medical solutions—from that year right through the COVID pandemic. Many years later during a 2014 tour of the CDC Museum in Atlanta, I shivered at the sight of an actual iron lung that used to encase the most unfortunate polio patients.

Dad's case wasn't an isolated occurrence. Each year in the early postwar period, polio crippled half a million people worldwide, including more than 35,000 Americans. In a White House speech, President Harry Truman said the fight against polio must be "total war in every city, town, and village throughout the land." The peak of the epidemic came in 1952 when more than 3,100 died in the United States alone. That might not sound like very high mortality compared to the millions of annual deaths from heart disease, cancer and, recently, COVID-19. But the nation was gripped with a fear of polio, perhaps because so many of its victims were children. Money and social status didn't protect people—even President Franklin Roosevelt had been stricken.

AN EARLY MEDICAL SOLUTION

Something else was happening in 1952. University of Pittsburgh virologist Jonas Salk began the first human tests of an inactivated poliovirus vaccine. His work built on two decades of research by others in New York and Boston. The project was funded by the National Foundation for Infantile Paralysis, commonly known as the March of Dimes. In April 1955, Salk announced the success of his field trials and urged all parents to be sure their children were vaccinated. I was soon lining up with classmates to receive my inoculation.

Despite assurances that the virus in Salk's vaccine was completely inactive, some parents held back out of a fear that the vaccine itself might cause the disease. Public health officials were frustrated because without widespread vaccination to create "herd immunity" in the population, polio would continue striking down thousands every year. Teenagers had been especially reluctant to get their shots. Then Elvis Presley came to the rescue.

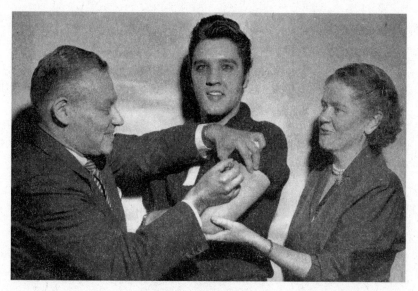

Elvis gets his polio shot.

My family and I were part of the millions of viewers who tuned in to CBS on Sunday nights for the *Ed Sullivan Show,* one of the most popular variety programs on American television. Elvis had recently become the top entertainer among US teenagers. Would the king of rock and roll agree to get a polio shot in front of press cameras while backstage before appearing on a live *Ed Sullivan* broadcast? He did, and within six months, the rate of teen vaccinations skyrocketed from less than 1 percent to more than 80 percent.*

---

* Much additional credit for the near-eradication of polio worldwide should go to Dr. Albert Sabin, whose oral vaccine—swallowed on a sugar cube—was licensed in the United States in 1961 and proved even more effective than Salk's injections. A true humanitarian, Sabin never patented his vaccine and received no royalties. He wanted the price to remain low so it would be available to everyone around the world.

ON WISCONSIN!

Even after an extraordinarily difficult childhood, Bernard Milken was never discouraged or bitter. My dad was determined to get a good education, despite a lack of funds and parental support. He applied to the University of Wisconsin at Madison where the tuition was so low—fifty-five dollars a year—he was able to pay for it by selling the Bulova watch he inherited from his father. It was a difficult decision to give up, one of the few remaining tangible links to his parents.

The Madison campus my mother described to me was shaped by natural beauty—rolling hills bookended lakes that hosted huge flocks of loons on their annual migrations. Among its stately buildings was a towering carillon with fifty-six bells that intoned Bach (and sometimes Jimmy Dorsey) with chimes on the hour. The campus was animated by student traditions—sledding down Baldwin Hill on cafeteria trays; homecoming bonfires; the mighty University of Wisconsin Marching Band playing "On Wisconsin!" at football games.

Unfortunately, Dad had little opportunity to enjoy these activities. He had to work at whatever jobs were available if he wanted to stay in school. One job was filling peanut machines around campus for a penny a bag; another was delivering newspapers. Later, when he was in law school, he worked as a waiter at the Phi Sigma Sigma sorority house.

Bernard's days brightened when a young woman named Ferne Zax joined Phi Sig. They fell in love and wanted to get married. But Ferne's father, Lou Zax, insisted she was too young and Bernard wasn't yet established in a stable career. He said they should wait a year. Everyone respected Lou—he'd been forced to take on major responsibilities early in life and was considered a good sounding board. So they postponed the nuptials.

During that year, Bernard moved to Chicago to work in an accounting firm and gain some on-the-job experience. On weekends, he drove back to Madison to see Ferne. Once the year had passed, they were married. Only a few days after the wedding, Dad sat for the three-day bar exam; and the day after that, they boarded the El Capitan train to Los Angeles, where they would have a fresh start. Ferne's aunt and uncle, Freda and Mo Singer, provided a bedroom until they could find their own apartment.

The Depression and World War II had made most Americans dependent on government. By the 1950s, however, cultural changes were instilling optimism in young couples. They told their kids they were part of a special generation and that one person could change the world. We could become anything we wanted and wouldn't need to be dependent on government.

In many ways, we reflected the 1950s values and ideals shown on such popular TV shows as *The Adventures of Ozzie and Harriett*. We were a close, happy family unit—my outgoing and creative mother, my industrious father, my brother Lowell, my sister Joni, and I. Financially, we were neither rich nor poor, just a typical middle-class family whose core tenets included charitable giving, community involvement, and learning. It wasn't all happiness, of course. For a couple of years, my mother made me take accordion lessons. To this day, the sound of an accordion evokes unpleasant memories!

Mom and Dad valued strong family and community ties. As this is written, my ninety-eight-year-old mother still prefers to live in the same house they bought more than seventy years ago.

My parents taught me about independence at a young age. When I was eight, they had shown me how to prepare trial balances for accounting clients. Then I began sorting checks and doing bank reconciliations. By age ten or eleven, I was working on income and cash-flow statements. Accounting became virtually another language to me. I began to appreciate the relationship between the financial numbers and the real world of people's businesses.

A LESSON FROM THE HORSES

The precision of accounting is far different from betting on horses. This is something I learned at age twelve. Dad's largest client was Desser and Garfield, a multistate property development firm. Among their many projects was an apartment complex in Del Mar, California, that happened to be near the Del Mar Thoroughbred Club "where the turf meets the surf." About a hundred miles south of our Encino home, it was a real showplace built by a group led by Bing Crosby. My dad needed to meet with some Del Mar–area clients and inspect their buildings, so he turned the trip into a mini-vacation for the family.

While Dad was working, my mother took me to the track, where she enjoyed betting on the horses. I was too young to wager, but Mom agreed to place a few bets for me. I launched into an exhaustive study of the thoroughbreds in search of some mathematical secret to winning. Three days of studying the tip sheets produced complete data on every horse. Then Mom placed my bets. By the end of the day, we just about broke even and all I had to show for my efforts was a headache. That's when I decided never to do that again. What a waste of time! There are far too many unpredictable factors to make sports betting a perfect science. Yet I was amazed that apparently intelligent people risked their hard-earned money on it. They used such frivolous criteria as the colors of the jockeys' silks and the sound of the horses' names.

A MORE IMPORTANT LESSON

I'll never forget our 1950s dinner table lessons. My parents often spoke about what constitutes success. It was drilled into us that success should not be measured in dollars; the truly successful person creates a family whose members are able to enjoy meaningful lives. And what gives life greater meaning is the opportunity to contribute to the community. Then Dad would lower his voice, as if to emphasize one final point: "No one in our society can have that unless *everyone* has a chance to achieve the American dream."

That had a profound effect on my thinking. Even today—whether I'm working on access to good healthcare, or to job opportunities, or to a COVID-19 vaccine—my Rosetta stone for policy development can be found in Dad's words: "No one can have a truly meaningful life unless *everyone* has a chance." The Milken Center for Advancing the American Dream in Washington, DC, is the most tangible expression my family can make to honor our parents.[*]

*　　　*　　　*

COMING OF AGE

Hesby Street Elementary School was small and nurturing. Birmingham Junior High and High School—a combined six-year institution—was gigantic and challenging. Originally built as an Army hospital during World War II, the school spread over a wide area with pathways connecting its multiple buildings. For many kids, the transition from sixth to seventh grade was like going from the kiddie wading pool into an Olympic swimming facility. I was in a "half-year class" that graduated from elementary school on a Friday in midwinter and started at Birmingham's intimidating campus— ten times larger than Hesby's—the next Monday.

Even though I was an outgoing, confident kid, my classmates and I hadn't fully appreciated what it would be like for a group of skinny

---

* See www.mcaad.org.

pre-teens to find themselves suddenly among other students who were as old as eighteen, a foot taller, and a hundred pounds heavier. We seventh graders were called "scrubs" and it was part of our fate to be "scrubbed" by high school bullies who smeared our faces with lipstick and deposited us—head first—into metal trash cans. One day, two heavyweights blocked my path as one of them sneered, "Where do you think you're going, scrub?" With that, he yanked the top off a tube of very red lipstick. Thinking fast, I blurted out, "Hey, I'm really good at math, I could help you with your homework." That feeble attempt at negotiating failed—I was soon upside down in a dark, smelly container.

I ran for class president, but lost. That's when I began to better understand the importance of communicating effectively with people who grew up in different circumstances from mine. Unlike Hesby Street School, where kids came from families with incomes ranging from the lower to upper middle-class, Birmingham had many students from very poor families. This heightened my awareness of social needs and provided motivation to work on community service projects. (After six years, I was the first recipient of the outstanding service award of the Encino Junior Chamber of Commerce.)

I'm thankful for my six years at Birmingham, which was unique among LA's public educational institutions. Its combined three years of junior high (now called middle school) with three years of high school was a big advantage, academically and socially. I was able to take advanced classes even in junior high. Before long, my academic progress in math moved so quickly that there were no more courses to take. I became a class of one and my teacher started giving me college-level work. I also enjoyed tutoring other kids.

One of my favorite activities at Birmingham was participating in the speech honor society, known as Gavel. I had represented Birmingham in Southern California Knowledge Bowl competitions

High School Senior Feted

VAN NUYS—Mike Milken, Birmingham High School senior, has received the first Outstanding Young Man Award presented by the Encino Junior Chamber of Commerce.

The award, an inscribed trophy, was presented at the recent senior class candlelight dinner at Sportsmen's Lodge.

Determination of the semiannual award is based on proven effective leadership, outstanding service rendered to school and community, acceptable academic achievement and desire for continued leadership and service.

A 1963 clipping from the Encino, California, newspaper.

that included oral questions testing recall, problem-solving, and critical thinking skills. Even more challenging were tournaments that required us to deliver prepared, extemporaneous, and impromptu speeches. Successful "imprompt" speakers had to be knowledgeable about many subjects because we weren't told the topic in advance, and there was little time to prepare. The organizer would announce your speech title and give you only seven minutes before you began speaking. No notes were permitted and of course there was no internet or nearby library. You had to have the information in your head. It helped that Mom and Dad had challenged me to speak confidently and defend my positions at the dinner table. Over the last sixty years, I've delivered thousands of speeches and impromptu talks. Thanks to early training, it's never a problem to organize my thoughts quickly and deliver them clearly.

Related to these activities were debate tournaments where two partners competed against other teams. My debate partner was my friend and later college roommate Greg Greenberg, who was even younger than I, and very bright. Starting in eighth grade, we participated in local debates after intensive preparation. Topics included foreign aid, education, civil rights, universal medical insurance, equal employment opportunity, and more. We spent long hours gathering facts, keeping up on the news, and organizing our research on index cards.

By ninth grade, we had qualified for a bigger contest—the regional tournament of the National Forensic League in Redlands, California. Dozens of schools from all over Southern California sent their best debaters and speakers. As the youngest team in the tournament, we faced stiff competition from other high school debate teams, many of them made up of twelfth graders.

During our tournament preparations that fall, we took time out to watch the 1960 presidential campaign debates pitting Vice President Richard Nixon against Senator John F. Kennedy. We evaluated their debate skills carefully and concluded that Nixon scored more points for content, but Kennedy won on presentation style.

The National Forensic League's debate topics that year were:

Resolved: The federal government should substantially increase regulation of labor unions; and *Resolved: The United Nations should be significantly strengthened.*

We spent weeks drawing up arguments on both sides of these questions. We wanted to have the whole picture, a complete understanding of whatever came up, readying not just our own positions, but every possible counter-position, and counters to those counters.

Greg and I traveled to schools all over Southern California taking on older kids. That didn't make us very popular. When we won second place in the Redlands tournament, one of the losing seniors sneered that we needed to get a life.*

---

* Decades later, when I was financing the nascent Cable News Network, CNN founder Ted Turner told me he had excelled in high school debates sponsored by the National Forensic League. So did Senator Bill Frist, a physician and former US Senate majority leader, when we discussed national health policies. We all had special memories of these events from our formative years. Supreme Court Justice Ketanji Brown Jackson also credits her

SPORTS

So many other extracurricular activities filled my days, it's a wonder there was time to study. Fortunately, I was a quick learner and never needed much sleep, even as a teenager. I was president of various service honor societies, a student government officer, an honor roll student, and a member of the tennis, track, and varsity basketball teams.

For a while, I thought there might be a real future for me in basketball. My growth spurt came early, making me one of the tallest kids in the ninth grade, when I made first team in the all-city league. At home, I practiced various kinds of shots to a hoop above the garage door. I tried dribbling blindfolded and wore ankle weights walking to the school bus because I thought it would help me jump higher.

Unfortunately, after ninth grade, I stopped growing. Over time, other players began to tower over me. My positions on the team went from center to forward to guard to spending a lot of time on the bench. At least I remained on the varsity as a sixth man.

(Later, when I arrived at college, I tried out for the freshman team. Watching me play, the coach said, "You're out of position." I explained my evolution from center to guard and asked him where I should be playing. He pointed to the stands and said, "You're going to be rooting for the team over there.")

Eventually, I was elected Birmingham High School's head cheerleader. (Back then, they called us "yell leaders.") This was considered

---

high school debate team experience with honing the oratorical skills that advanced her legal career. These days, when I'm talking to our grandchildren, I carry on my parents' dinner table tradition by encouraging them to expound on their ideas clearly. And they now participate in their own school debate programs.

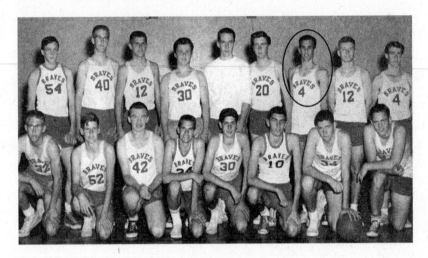

On the Birmingham High basketball team.

a leadership position in which you represented the entire school with great energy and spirit. I worked hard at it and like to think I played some small role in Birmingham football winning the city title that year in front of thousands of fans. But I was no more enthusiastic in leading the cheers for Birmingham than my dad was in rooting for Wisconsin Badgers football.

On New Year's Day 1963, when I was in eleventh grade, we settled in to watch the Badgers on television. That year's Rose Bowl game pitted the top-ranked USC Trojans against number two Wisconsin for the national championship. Years later, the *Los Angeles Times* called it the most memorable Rose Bowl in history. As the final quarter began, USC led 42–14 and gloom pervaded our living room. Then Wisconsin's quarterback, Ron Vander Kelen went to work, leading the team in scoring twenty-three unanswered points. The neighbors must have wondered what all the cheering was about. Wisconsin was on a roll, but as time ran out, they came up just short, 42–37. Even in losing, Vander Kelen was named most valuable player.

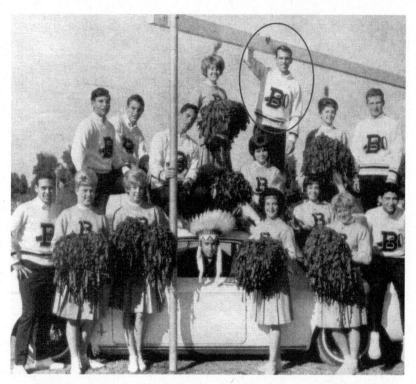

As the head cheerleader. Future actress Sally Field is in front of me.

LORI

One of the highlights of my years at Birmingham was meeting Lori Hackel in Mr. Ramirez's seventh-grade social studies class. She didn't know what to make of me since I had a reputation for being outspoken—always raising my hand and challenging the teachers. In contrast, Lori was more restrained and probably considered my academic enthusiasm a bit unseemly. Perhaps I was attracted to her precisely because we had different temperaments.

We started dating in ninth grade (carefully chaperoned by parents).

Although I was voted "Most Spirited" and "Friendliest" in our high school class, it was Lori who earned the honor "Most Likely to Succeed." During our senior year, she was elected a prom princess and I was the prom king. We've been together more than sixty-four years, and she will always be my princess.

THREE

College and the Real World

Leadership in high school gave me confidence about the future. I narrowed the choice of possible colleges to two: the California Institute of Technology (Caltech) and the University of California–Berkeley. Some of my friends who graduated from MIT will disagree, but I considered Caltech the world's top scientific school. Given my interests in math and science, it was a logical choice. But with its much smaller faculty and student body, Caltech would have locked me into a narrower path. Berkeley had an unparalleled breadth of academics, giving students more freedom to switch majors if their interests changed. It had been rated the number-one undergraduate and graduate institution, and there was a sense that you could see the entire world from the corner of Bancroft Way and Telegraph Avenue.

When Berkeley accepted my application, I looked forward to studying at a university whose faculty included many Nobel laureates in science. It also seemed to me that I was well prepared for such an internationally sophisticated environment. I'd followed news events closely—Sputnik, the space race, the 1960 election, the Bay of Pigs invasion, the Cuban Missile Crisis, and the growing civil rights movement.

In August 1963, I was moved when watching on television as Martin Luther King Jr. delivered his "I Have a Dream" speech in front of the Lincoln Memorial. It wasn't just Dr. King's soaring eloquence— it was the way he captured the essence of the American dream.

One Friday morning just six weeks before my January 1964 graduation, I heard static on the school's public address system. *Must be a fire drill*, I thought. That wouldn't be so bad—it was a nice day and it would be good to get outside. The wall clock said 11:08.

It wasn't a fire drill. "I'm very sorry to announce," the principal's somber voice began, "that John F. Kennedy, president of the United States, was shot this morning in Dallas, Texas. At eleven o'clock (1:00 p.m. Central Time), just a few minutes ago, he was pronounced dead." A collective gasp and a few fearful shrieks in our classroom drowned out the rest of the announcement. It was something about classes being canceled.

Everyone returned home in shock. What I noticed, however, was the different ways this cataclysmic event affected people. Some classmates wept and said how sad it was that such a wonderful man had died in the prime of life. What concerned me was how, after the assassinations of three previous presidents—Lincoln, Garfield, and McKinley—there hadn't been enough security to protect Kennedy. Was this something bigger? Something that could threaten our democracy? Who was behind it? What was the motive? Would the country rally around the vice president?

That night, I went to temple with other students. It was difficult to concentrate on the outpouring of grief and tributes to the fallen leader. My mind kept returning to the other questions. One thing seemed clear: The happy society of my youth would never be the same.

THE FIRST BABY BOOMERS

My unusual January graduation meant there was only a weekend to transition from high school to college. Over that weekend, I would travel from LA to Berkeley, move into the Bancroft Dorms, and prepare for the new term's classes. As a seventeen-year-old born in 1946, I was among the first of the baby boomers going off to college. Our cohort had been—and would continue to be—part of transformational social and cultural changes throughout our lives.

My dorm roommate was my former Birmingham debate partner, Greg Greenberg. That fall, during my second semester, I pledged at the Sigma Alpha Mu (ΣAM) fraternity known as "Sammy." Its mission of "instilling strong fraternal values, offering social and service opportunities, encouraging academic excellence and teaching leadership skills" appealed to me. Soon, I was elected president of the freshman pledge class—twenty-two guys who were almost all high achievers.

As with most fraternities, there were hazing rituals, but the skills I had developed by leading high school organizations helped me deal with the upperclassmen. I welcomed this additional challenge. As pledge class president, I had to be part team leader, part advocate for my pledge brothers, and part psychologist. Despite their earlier high school distinction—many had been student body presidents or valedictorians—some found it difficult to cope with Berkeley's wide-open culture and fraternity hazing. One started crying when he was ordered to do push-ups or clean toilets or some other menial task. "Hey, don't worry about it," I told him. "This isn't real; they're just playing mind games with you. Do what they tell you and it will soon be over."

Berkeley put everything—good and bad—at your disposal. That was fine if you were mature enough to handle it. But it could be difficult for emotionally immature or insecure people. I remember one fraternity brother who was the greatest athlete I've ever known. He was a few classes behind mine at Birmingham and set many school records. The fastest runner in track, he once scored thirty points against the top basketball team in LA. In baseball, his batting average was close to .400 and as a pitcher, he threw a shutout in the city championship. He was a hot prospect for the Major League Baseball draft and I have no doubt he would have had a fabulous professional career. Other than sports, however, he wasn't sure what to do with his life. He finally decided to follow several of his older friends who had gone to Berkeley, which granted him a full athletic scholarship.

This fraternity brother seemed to have it all, except for one thing: the security of a stable family. During his sophomore year, his parents divorced; he seemed confused and eventually disappeared. My repeated attempts to find him were unsuccessful. Even today, I wonder if he would have been better able to face the pressures of professional sports than to deal with the stresses of Berkeley's wide-open environment at a time of cultural upheaval. I sometimes think about this when managing diverse groups of people who respond to job pressures differently.

FREE SPEECH

Soon after I joined Sammy, the Free Speech Movement erupted on campus. This was no minor demonstration—it was ground zero for 1960s student activism, a massive revolutionary outcry in the vanguard of uprisings across the country and eventually the world.

Following the tactics of the civil rights movement and foreshadowing the Vietnam War protests, Free Speech leaders Mario Savio, Jack Weinberg, and others inspired thousands of students. They protested a ban on campus political activities including any publication that wasn't "approved" by the administration. Eventually, they forced the university to reverse the ban and acknowledge the right of all students to free speech. That included political activities and the right to publish the student newspaper without interference. Now, just as I had with the Kennedy assassination, I tried to place the campus disruptions in a broader social context.

Berkeley had always tolerated diverse views. That's one reason I chose to go there. Anyone with a cause could set up a card table on Bancroft Way to distribute propaganda: the American Communist Party on one side, a Nazi group across from them, the ever-popular Sexual Freedom League, and dozens of others from all over the world. After the Free Speech Movement succeeded in wringing some concessions from the university, more advocacy groups set up tables. The creative ferment was energizing.

While all this was going on, I was leading a pledge class that

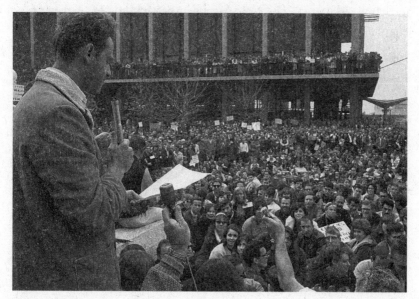

Mario Savio leads a free speech demonstration at Berkeley in December of 1964.

reflected the same diversity of views found in the broad university community. The demonstrations were almost all peaceful and enjoyed the overwhelming support of the student body. I knew some of the leaders, including Mario Savio, and thought there's no reason for him not to speak out if he felt he could change the world.

Berkeley students took pride in their forbearance of even extreme opinions. One day, the leader of the American Nazi Party, George Lincoln Rockwell, appeared on campus to speak in the school gym. The administration was quite concerned because he had stirred up riots at other campuses. Rockwell started spouting off about white supremacy, which he justified by claiming that white people had bigger brain cavities. He said that provided more room for your brain to expand. Instead of rioting, everyone just laughed at him. It was absurd.

Events were unfolding with breathtaking speed. Martin Luther King Jr. and more than seven hundred of his followers were arrested in Selma, Alabama. The Cold War was getting hotter. A new president promised sweeping changes in a "Great Society." Within the year, he signed the landmark Civil Rights Act of 1964. The next year, the Voting Rights Act of 1965 aimed to overcome state and local barriers to the franchise. When the United States began heavy bombing of North Vietnam in 1965, anti-war protests began in earnest.

Berkeley was in the center of it all.

*   *   *

WATTS: THE ROOTS OF DESPAIR

After three semesters at Berkeley, I thought I'd seen everything. My interactions with students from every social sector, years of following the news, and debate tournament preparations had made me well aware of widespread discrimination against racial and religious minority groups. I knew how fortunate I was compared to relatives who never left Europe and were killed in the Holocaust. I'd watched in disgust as nightly TV reports showed police and attack dogs assaulting peaceful demonstrators in southern states. Growing up in Los Angeles, however, I'd never personally felt discrimination. I retained an idealist's view that America was a land of opportunity, especially in this city of dreams, the place where movies were made. It seemed almost self-evident that anyone with ambition could get ahead.

That belief was destroyed when I returned to Los Angeles to work through the 1965 summer break. August 11, the Watts Riots broke out a few miles from our Encino home. Watts is in South Central Los Angeles, an area I knew well having joined my father on calls to his accounting clients, some of whom owned small manufacturing businesses. Even when I was quite young, he let me ask them all kinds of questions: How do you run your business? Where does the money come from to start a business? How do you train employees? Speaking with men and women who owned these community businesses was a good learning experience.

I'd competed in high school speech tournaments in South Central, attended sporting events, there and tutored younger kids. It was hard to understand why the residents of this area were burning their own community. Yet the rioting was so extensive that the LA Rams–Dallas Cowboys preseason football game at the Los Angeles Coliseum was postponed for three days. Dad, Lowell, and I went to the game and I have to admit it seemed strange to be watching football when buildings were still smoldering within blocks of the stadium. Sitting in the half-filled stands, we could hear police and fire sirens. You didn't need to go to Vietnam to see military personnel carriers—they were patrolling the streets of Los Angeles.

Driving home, my father noted how unusual it was to have a game with no touchdowns—the Rams won 9–0 on three field goals. But my mind wasn't on football. When we got home that night, I said, "Dad, I'm going down to Watts tomorrow to see for myself what's really going on." My father was aghast. "I hope you've come into an inheritance, because if you do that, you'll need it to pay for the rest of college on your own." I thought, or at least hoped, he was joking because I'd already decided to go.

The next morning, I told my mother I needed to run some errands, got in my blue Ford Falcon, and drove south on the just completed 405 Freeway. Parking as close as the National Guard troops would allow, I walked the rest of the way. Several nights of rioting had created a desolate moonscape of destruction. Fires still flared up in some places. The smoke stung my eyes and caught in my throat. Block after block had been reduced to rubble. *Why*, I asked myself, *would the people who live here torch their own community?* Eventually, I came upon an African American man in front of the burned-out shell of a small factory. He was just staring at it.

We talked for a few minutes, and he told me this was the place where he worked. Rioters had set fire to it and although he didn't participate, he did nothing to stop them. In fact, he yelled encouragement. It seemed unbelievable. Here was a man who said he had a family and now he was without a job. I asked why he'd made no effort to save his only source of income. He looked at me as if I were from another planet (and in a sense, I was). "It's not *my* business," he said. "Some white guy by the ocean owns it. Negroes like me don't own nothing." He explained that his father had worked for years hoping to open a similar small factory. But he always felt like an outsider and no bank would give the older man the financing needed to get it started. "He couldn't get a loan. I can't get a loan. There's nothing to hope for."

Suddenly I realized that all the civil rights laws, all the urban

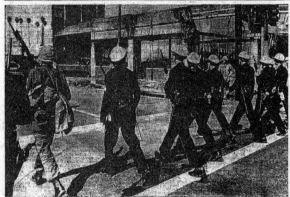

The Watts Riots increased my awareness of social disparities and became a turning point in my life.

reconstruction projects, all the student demonstrations, wouldn't achieve social justice if there was no access to capital. It was the essential missing piece.

DEMOCRATIZING CAPITAL

At Berkeley, I'd witnessed the Free Speech Movement and other forms of student dissent. This was different. Now I saw the actual roots of despair. That man in Watts described the factory where he'd earned his paycheck as "theirs," not "his." I began to understand that success in America requires access to opportunity, which almost always requires access to financial capital. This man had neither, and he wasn't alone.

It all seemed so unfair, so antithetical to the concept of the American dream.

A few years later, the *Report of the National Advisory Commission on Civil Disorders* said the riots that began in Watts and spread to other cities were a result of "structural racism." It concluded that "white institutions created it, white institutions maintain it and white society condones it." I never denied the terrible legacy of segregation, but neither was I ready to accept that "white society condones it." Sure, there were plenty of bigots, but I believed that most right-thinking people wanted a more inclusive society. I wanted to help build that society.

Other Berkeley students were sincere in pursuing civil rights as they led the social upheavals of the mid-1960s. But I began to see that civil rights—the great and worthy cause of my generation's youth—meant more than the right to sit up front in a bus or eat at a lunch counter. It meant more than the right to attend a good school or merely hold a job. It also meant the right to participate in economic society through *ownership*.

My best chance to help change things for the better seemed to be in finance, an area where it looked like I could continue to develop useful skills. My father had given me a good start in accounting. That led to a part-time job during high school with a local professional investor, Herman Fishman, who introduced me to the rudiments of securities research. I also learned a few things about manufacturing from a friend and client of Dad's, Harvey Cooper; he owned Maxine of Hollywood, a business that made women's swimwear. Now I was determined to build on the base of those experiences and turn them into something socially useful—the democratization of capital.

Returning to campus two weeks later, I switched my major to

finance and business in the belief that economic liberty should go hand in hand with political liberty. The freedom to own and build a business—a business that would create jobs in the community— seemed as important as the freedom to cast a vote.*

THE DEMOCRATIZATION OF OPPORTUNITY

Changing my major—giving up plans to be a scientist, maybe even an astronaut—was a wrenching decision. But after everything I'd experienced, I reevaluated my goals and was ready to set off in a new direction.

One afternoon, I came across an interesting paper by a young economist named Gary Becker. The gist of it was that people don't always act rationally, the way economic models predict. It helped me understand why a man in Watts would feel so much rage about an unfair economic system that he would do things that were contrary to his own interests. Gary and I became friends in the late 1970s. In 1992, he won the Nobel Prize in Economics for his theories of human capital.

Late in his career, Gary was involved in many of our efforts at the Milken Institute's Center for Financial Markets and at our *Faster-Cures* center. We often shared the stage at the annual Milken Institute Global Conference. After he died, I was honored to speak at a memorial for him at the University of Chicago.

Gary once explained irrationality to me: "Rationally, you know that cigarettes are bad for you. But if you were a student in the 1960s, it could seem rational to smoke because (a) it seems cool—a route to

---

* I made a related point in 1989 when I delivered a speech to the Conference of Black Mayors: They were gaining increasing political power, but recent legislation had effectively restricted lending in many cities and states with large numbers of African Americans.

social acceptance and a showing of independence from disapproving parents, combined with (b) a belief, no matter how misguided, that science will have figured out a cure for lung cancer before it develops in you." That kind of iconoclastic thinking helped make Gary such a delight to his friends and students.

THE JOURNAL OF
POLITICAL ECONOMY

Volume LXX   FEBRUARY 1962   Number 1

IRRATIONAL BEHAVIOR AND ECONOMIC THEORY[1]

GARY S. BECKER
Columbia University

I. INTRODUCTION

ALTHOUGH it has long been agreed that traditional economic theory "assumes" rational behavior, at one time there was considerable disagreement over the meaning of the word "rational." To many, the word suggested

of a well-ordered function, such as a utility or profit function.

Strong and even violent differences developed, however, at a different level. Critics claim that households and firms do not maximize, at least not consistently, that preferences are not well ordered,

Early in his career, Gary's innovations in economics were considered as controversial by establishment economists as my later innovations in finance were by establishment bankers. He believed that market-based solutions, not government handouts, would provide the greatest social opportunity for the disadvantaged. I believed that market-centered access to capital, not institutionally controlled banking relationships, would provide the greatest growth opportunity for entrepreneurs.

THEORY VS. REALITY

My new major in business proved to be just as data-intensive as math and science. I was fortunate to have access to CRSP tapes—

records of stock prices compiled on magnetic tapes by the Center for Research in Security Prices at the University of Chicago. The tapes ran on massive room-sized computers. Back then, these giant machines incorporated the very latest in technology, although they had millions of times less capacity than today's mobile phones. I was introduced to the basics of programming using IBM punched cards, an old paper-based system first introduced in 1928. (Remarkably, these cards are still used in some rural US voting machines.)

As part of my research about credit I obtained a book that would change my life. It was called *Corporate Bond Quality and Investor Experience* by W. Braddock Hickman. It was far from a bestseller, which is not surprising since most people would have found it deadly dull—hundreds of pages filled with dense text, even-denser footnotes, yield charts, and tables of default rates for bonds issued by railroads, utilities, and industrial companies between 1900 and 1943. Scanning the columns, however, I sensed a previously undiscovered pattern—a disparity between theory and reality.

Standard financial theory says there's a straight-line correlation between risk and return. The market provides a higher yield on investments that seem to carry a higher risk. Investors supposedly do equally well in low-yield or high-yield securities because the market makes a risk adjustment. The high-yield investor will collect more from each issuer that makes its promised interest payments, but the total amount he receives will be no more than the low-yield investor's steadier return because some issuers will miss payments.

That's the theory. But what I saw in Hickman's book told me the theory was wrong because the market had historically overestimated the risk of higher-yielding investments. He summarized the main conclusion of his study—a period that included World War I and the Great Depression:

Corporate Bond Quality
and
Investor Experience

BY W. BRADDOCK HICKMAN

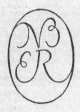

A STUDY BY THE
NATIONAL BUREAU OF ECONOMIC RESEARCH, NEW YORK

PUBLISHED BY
PRINCETON UNIVERSITY PRESS, PRINCETON
1958

On the average and over long periods, the life-span yields realized on high-grade bonds were below those on low-grade bonds, with the result that investors, in the aggregate, obtained better returns on the low grades . . . the higher promised returns exacted on the low grades at offering proved to be more than sufficient to offset the higher default losses.

That conclusion got me interested in studying the history of credit. I discovered that high-yield bonds had been an important economic tool for hundreds of years: The Dutch East India Company had issued them early in the seventeenth century to finance their activities around the world; the Massachusetts Bay Colony sold bonds paying a high interest rate before America had a constitution; the first US

Treasury secretary, Alexander Hamilton, financed the growth of the young nation with high-yield debt; America's nineteenth-century railroads could not have been built without selling these kinds of bonds to European investors; and J. P. Morgan used high-yield bonds to finance the creation of U.S. Steel.

After studying this history and many other reference materials, I wrote down six principles of credit:[*]

1. Credit is what counts, not leverage.

2. Interest rates are never predictable over time.

3. Ratings are a poor predictor of credit quality across industrial sectors.

4. Risks in sovereign and government debt have long been underestimated.

5. Real estate loans are rarely high-quality investments.

6. The value of debt securities underpins all capital markets.

It wasn't long before I concluded that much of what my professors were saying, and what the textbooks reported, was simply wrong. For example, they said that sovereign debt—a financial obligation of governments—was a safer investment than corporate debt. It didn't take much digging for me to find many examples of government bond defaults. Some countries routinely issued bonds every twenty years or so, later stopped paying interest, and couldn't return the principal. Yet supposedly sophisticated investors lined up to buy their next issuance. It made no sense.

This took me back to my childhood when I'd quiz my parents' guests

---

[*] A more detailed explanation of these six points is in my article "Components of Prosperity" at www.mikemilken.com.

at their Saturday night bridge parties. I was shocked then to discover they didn't know the answers; and now some of these esteemed professors at a great university were poorly informed about the history of credit. In fairness, it wasn't just the academics. In future years I learned that many business CEOs, financiers, and government leaders—even treasury secretaries and Federal Reserve chairmen—were often just as ignorant of the facts uncovered in my studies of credit history.

The Formula

During my undergraduate studies, a set of ideas about society, finance, and prosperity began to coalesce in my mind. Three types of assets—human capital, social capital, and financial capital—were much more closely related than most people realized. Without social capital—schools, for example—human capital can't develop. And without human capital—people's skills—financial capital can't be deployed productively. I expressed these ideas in a formula:

$$P=\Sigma Ft_i*(\Sigma HC_i+\Sigma SC_i+\Sigma RA_i)$$

This formula says that *prosperity* in any society equals the effect of *financial technologies* acting as a multiplier on the total value of *human capital, social capital,* and the *real assets* on balance sheets.

"Human capital" means the collective value of people's abilities, training, and experience. It's the most valuable resource on earth.*

---

* I've often illustrated the importance of human capital by citing examples of how one person can make a big difference. Consider the case of two companies, Sony and Apple. Sony was founded and led for half a century by Akio Morita, a brilliant businessman who built an enterprise synonymous with technology innovation and quality. By 1997, Sony's market value was $34 billion, more than twenty times greater than the $1.65 billion of Apple, then an also-ran in the computer business. In 1997, not long before Morita-san died, Apple rehired Steve Jobs. As this is written in October 2022, Apple's $2.30 trillion market capitalization is more than twenty-eight times greater than Sony's $80.8 billion. Their relative values shifted by a factor greater than five hundred sixty.

Societies that achieve the greatest lasting prosperity are those that include all citizens in building human capital. When everyone has access to education, can participate in the political process, and can aspire to ownership of property, stable economic growth is most likely to follow. This explains why countries like South Korea, Japan, and Singapore—with few natural resources—enjoy multiples of the per capita incomes of such resource-rich nations as Mexico, Brazil, and Nigeria.

"Social capital" includes universal education and healthcare, police and fire protection, religious freedom, a sense of neighborhood bonds and widely available cultural resources. It also includes the incentives for risk-taking inherent in established property rights, protection of creditors, regulatory continuity, transparent markets, and rigorous financial reporting standards.

"Real assets" are cash, receivables, real estate, factories, capital equipment, and anything else that can be assigned a specific current value. They're what you see on the left side of a company's balance sheet.

"Financial technology" refers to new processes and organizational forms, innovative types of securities or derivatives of securities, and new ways of bringing investors together with sources of capital. Very little financial technology existed when I was a student.

I've revisited my prosperity formula over the years and never found reason to change the equation. It remains my core understanding of the relationship between finance and a healthy society. It also led me to new thinking about finance in a larger context. It was clear that

---

One person can also make a big difference in sports. During the 1978–79 basketball season, the Boston Celtics won only twenty-nine games and finished last in their division. Over the next twelve years, they averaged more than twice as many wins—sixty-one per season—and made the playoffs every year, including three world championships. The difference was Larry Bird, a twelve-time All-Star, who played for the Celtics from 1980 through 1991. Then there's Michael Jordan, often called the greatest basketball player of all time. In 1984, the year before Jordan joined the Chicago Bulls, home game attendance totaled 261,000. Five years into his career, attendance had grown to 737,000.

the true value of a business (or, for that matter, of a household or a country) is often not fully reflected in the audited numbers, which ignore human and social capital.*

My studies at Berkeley showed that access to financial capital—the lifeblood of business—has been severely restricted throughout history. Even in the 1960s, it was still controlled by relatively few bankers who doled it out to privileged clients—the several hundred corporations that boasted an "investment-grade" rating. As one of the most regulated industries in the nation, banks were encouraged and predisposed to provide loans only to "safe" borrowers and their managements, who almost invariably were male, white, and "established."

This served to institutionalize the routine denial of capital to entrepreneurs with great business ideas but no establishment credentials. Among its many victims were minorities and women. Marginalized and disenfranchised, it was easy for them to believe *this* America wasn't *their* America and that there was no economic way to make it so. In *their* America, capital wasn't democratic and therefore neither was prosperity.

*   *   *

Eventually, I laid out five career goals in finance:

1. Democratize capital so aspiring entrepreneurs had access to thousands of investors—not just a few large banks—in expanding their businesses and promoting job growth.

2. Establish research as the foundation for financial markets.

---

* One business that does list human capital on the balance sheet is professional sports, where players' contracts show up under liabilities. Of course, these numbers are not always an accurate reflection of a player's value. A talented rookie might have a relatively small salary while an over-the-hill veteran could have a contract specifying payments far in excess of his real added value.

PROSPERITY FORMULA

$$P=\Sigma Ft_i{}^*(\Sigma HC_i+\Sigma SC_i+\Sigma RA_i)$$

Financial Technology	Human Capital	Social Capital	Real Assets
Innovative processes & components including: • Convertible bonds • Preferred stock • High-yield bonds • Collateralized loans • Collateralized bonds • Equity-linked securities • Securitized obligations (mortgages, credit cards, etc.) • Derivatives	Productivity: • Skills • Education • Training • Experience • Creativity • Habits • Values	• Rule of law • Property rights • Public health • Universal education • Religious freedom • Police/fire protection • Cultural resources • Universal suffrage • Protection of creditors • Rigorous financial reporting standards • Transparent markets • Regulatory continuity • Environmental protection	• Cash • Receivables • Real estate • Factories • Capital equipment • Roads • Buildings • Infrastructure • Natural resources

3. Create new balance-sheet structures that better matched the corporate environment of each company with its industry, financial markets, economy, regulation, and society.

4. More closely align the incentives of owners and managers.

5. Diversify risk by pooling and securitizing various assets.

Over the next twenty years, with the help of thousands of colleagues, customers, and competitors, each of these goals was achieved.

SOME EXTRA PIZZA

In one of my last semesters at Berkeley, I signed up for linear algebra in economics, sometimes called the university's most difficult course. It involved mathematical modeling of the real world using dense, almost incomprehensible equations. Most students who took the course hated it. I loved it. It helped me formulate my ideas of how you build an economy and a functioning society with all the complex interactions involved. Soon I was relating classroom theories back to actual experiences, including what I'd observed as a little kid helping my father balance his clients' books.

It wasn't all studying, of course. We had plenty of good times at the fraternity house (including some foolish shenanigans reminiscent of the movie *Animal House*). Eventually, I became the fraternity's exchequer (treasurer) and then the prior (president). All of us at Sammy were close and a number of us still keep in touch.

One of my happiest days on campus was when Lori Hackel, the love of my life, transferred there from UC Santa Barbara. She pledged, and later became president of, the Alpha Epsilon Phi sorority. In our senior year, she headed Berkeley's largest sorority and I headed the largest fraternity.

I planned to propose to her on Valentine's Day, 1968. A fancy restaurant would have been nice for such an important occasion, but after years of dating and saving up for a ring, there wasn't enough money left for an extravagant meal. We went to Giovanni's Italian Pizza, which was close by and cheap. The plain cheese pizza I ordered for the two of us didn't satisfy my hearty appetite. Then I noticed the people at the next table were on their way out the door, leaving half an extra-large pizza loaded with toppings. Trying to be as casual as possible, I inched my chair over and rescued the remainders before the busboy came to clear it.

"What are you doing?" Lori whispered. Her eyes flitted around the restaurant in apparent embarrassment. But she was also laughing.

Later, when we were alone in my car, I asked her to marry me. She then asked me to get on my knees in the compact Falcon—no easy task. Somehow, I pushed the driver's seat all the way back, squeezed down on the floor behind the steering wheel and put the ring on her finger. I got up, she slid across the bench seat, and we kissed. With my arm around her shoulders, we drove back to the sorority house.

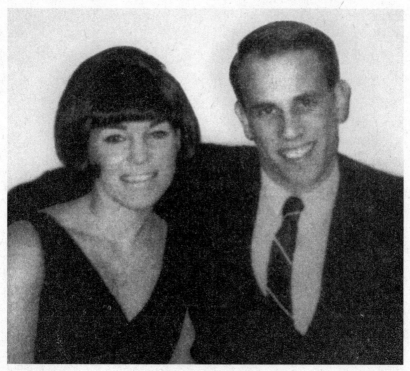

Lori and me in 1968.

FOUR

Clinical Trials

_____

Those of us who lived through 1968 share vivid memories and, for some, a sense that the social structure was unraveling. Early in the year, the Tet Offensive signaled a major escalation of the Vietnam War. In April, Martin Luther King Jr., who had inspired so many of us, fell to an assassin's bullet. Beginning in May, France was virtually shut down by riots, general strikes, and university occupations. During the Democratic National Convention in Chicago that August, the city erupted with violent clashes between anti-war protesters and police.

Another event that profoundly affected me, and the nation, occurred just a few blocks from my office on Wilshire Boulevard in Los Angeles. Having completed most of my undergraduate course requirements, I didn't need to be on campus for the final quarter as long as I showed up to take the final exams. It was an opportunity to earn some money for graduate school before the wedding. I resumed what had previously been a summer job with Touche Ross & Company, then one of the largest accounting firms.* I was working more than a hundred hours a week, but took an hour off to vote in California's June 4 presidential primary election, won by Senator Robert F. Kennedy.

The next day, a friend who worked on Kennedy's campaign invited me to join him at the nearby Ambassador Hotel, where the senator was scheduled to speak that evening. I considered attending, but decided against it because of a looming work deadline. A few minutes after midnight on June 5, Kennedy was mortally wounded by a lone gunman, Sirhan Sirhan. It was easy to approach the senator as he departed through the hotel kitchen. In those days, presidential candidates had no Secret Service protection. Kennedy had only two bodyguards, one of whom was former professional football star Roosevelt Grier, now my friend and colleague at the Milken Family Foundation. That night, Rosey had been assigned to protect Ethel Kennedy, the senator's wife. When he heard shots, he ran forward, grabbed Sirhan's gun and wrestled him to the floor.

The combined impact of all these 1968 events created a sense in people across the land that no one was truly safe. Three admired leaders, the two Kennedys and Martin Luther King Jr., were struck down in less than five years. For Lori and me, it cast a pall over otherwise joyous preparations for our summer wedding. The two killings that spring also increased a sense of urgency about getting on with my personal mission. With memories of the Watts Riots a few years earlier, I was more determined than ever to work for social change.

---

* Touche Ross was one of the "Big 8" accounting organizations at the time. (After consolidations, the industry now has a "Big 4.") As I worked in their Los Angeles office during 1967 and 1968, the smartest manager I encountered was a woman. What I didn't understand was why she wasn't a partner like many of her male colleagues, who struck me as less qualified. When I raised this issue with Neil Bersch, the managing partner of the LA office, he explained that it wasn't their policy to have female partners. Two decades later, I was happy to be able to finance the first woman to acquire a Fortune 500 company she hadn't inherited.

GRAD SCHOOL

The wedding in Los Angeles was on August 11, coincidentally three years to the day from the start of the riots. After a honeymoon in Hawaii, Lori and I headed east. The first stop was Chicago to visit my maternal grandparents even though we knew the city would be under siege because of expected anti-war protests. Soon we arrived in Philadelphia, where I had enrolled in the graduate MBA program at the University of Pennsylvania's Wharton School of Business.

Wharton was expensive, but it helped that they had accepted my application for a Joseph Wharton Fellowship. These are awarded to students with "outstanding records of academic, personal, and professional accomplishments." Even with the fellowship, earnings from jobs, and help from parents, our finances were very tight. Each night after dinner, we wrote down every penny spent that day. Instead of urban Philadelphia's expensive housing, we found a small apartment near a train station in the village of Ridley Park, about ten miles south of the Penn campus.

Most mornings, we'd commute to 30th Street Station. From there, I walked to my classes. There was a trolley that covered the dozen blocks faster, but walking saved a forty-five-cent fare. Lori would take the Market Street subway downtown to her job as a buyer at Lit Brothers department store. Lit positioned itself as a moderately priced alternative to the more upscale John Wanamaker emporium.

WALL STREET'S PAPER BLIZZARD

After studying credit at Berkeley and working at Touche Ross, I was ready for a more rigorous and specialized study of capital structure—

how companies manage their balance sheets.* I had chosen Wharton because it was a step in the direction of achieving my five financial career goals.

Wharton allowed me to sign up for three majors—operations research, information systems, and finance—while waiving some other course requirements because of my prior study and knowledge. I was happy to have the opportunity to advance my career plan and to show that finance could make a positive difference. It was a chance to test the academic theories I'd developed as an undergraduate.

Some of my Berkeley friends had joined the Peace Corps, entered law school, worked on Capitol Hill or followed any of a dozen other worthy pursuits that might contribute to social progress. I had determined that the financial community could also effect change. After all, it was the gatekeeper of investment capital that allowed businesses to create jobs, and it seemed to me the gate wasn't open wide enough.

My professors soon learned that I was very serious about capital access. Just as I had challenged my parents' bridge-party guests when I was eight years old, as well as my high school and college teachers, now I was asking tough questions about finance. Years later, my favorite Wharton professor, Morris Mendelson, paid me a compliment by saying that I improved teaching because the professors had to be especially well-prepared if I was in their class.

I was always closer to the faculty and PhD candidates than to my fellow MBA students. Morris and I remained friends for the rest of his life. A few months into my first year at Wharton, he reached

---

* In the 1990s, I had friendly debates with Nobel laureate Merton Miller about the importance of capital structure—whether it had a significant impact on long-term corporate success. Merton had coauthored the well-known Modigliani-Miller theorem, which posited that the relative levels of debt and equity made little difference. My view is that this ratio fundamentally affects the cost of capital and often the very survival of an enterprise.

out to me with an intriguing proposition. He and many others were getting concerned about the growing "back-office" problem on Wall Street. Whenever a customer traded a security, the brokerage had to record the transaction in the customer's account and mail a confirmation slip. The buying and selling brokers exchanged checks and physically delivered the securities, often to a distant city. That had been the process since the eighteenth century. Yet the volume of trades made each day's transactions a paperwork nightmare. Investors grumbled about their brokers' errors and the newspapers called it "Wall Street's Meltdown." The New York Stock Exchange finally had to shorten trading hours so member firms could keep up with the flood of paper. Eventually the entire stock exchange closed down every Wednesday.

Professor Mendelson suggested how I might help a local Philadelphia-based firm confront these issues by making good use of my newly acquired knowledge of operations research and information systems. He introduced me to what was then considered the leading equities research firm, Drexel Harriman Ripley, where I accepted a consulting job offer. As a public school–educated Californian from a Jewish family, I didn't fit the mold of this "white shoe" firm's usual recruits. But I established close relationships with three of Drexel's senior managers—Paul Miller, Clay Anderson, and Jay Sherrerd—who later launched a highly successful investment management firm based on fundamental research. They agreed to publish my Berkeley research about credit if I would work on the immediate back-office delivery and operations problems.*

Drexel published my credit work in May 1970 just as my MBA class was graduating. The firm then offered me a full-time job as assistant to the CEO at what seemed like an astronomical salary of $25,000 a year plus bonus. The timing was good because Lori was

---

* When Miller, Anderson, and Sherrerd left Drexel, they were succeeded by coheads of research Tom Beach and Ernie Whitman, who published my research.

about to give up her job and enroll at Penn's Graduate School of Education to study for a master's degree.

Lori and I had moved just east of the Delaware River to a highrise called Landmark Apartments in Cherry Hill, New Jersey, where there was a convenient new high-speed transit line to downtown Philadelphia. A few months later, however, my commute went in the other direction when I took a "temporary" assignment in Drexel's New York office as head of fixed income research. I was twenty-four years old.

A LONG COMMUTE

Very early each morning, I'd drive one exit on Interstate 295 to the bus station in Mount Laurel, New Jersey; then take a Trailways bus to the Port Authority Bus Terminal on West Forty-Second Street in New York. From there, the A train ran down the west side of Manhattan to the Fulton Street station in the financial district. Then I'd walk about six blocks lugging bags of financial documents to the office at 60 Broad Street. I can't say that part of it was enjoyable, especially when it was raining or snowing; and it was a long haul—five hours roundtrip—but I got lots of work done in transit.

The only problem with this routine was when someone would take the seat next to me on the bus and strike up a conversation. I like people—after all, I had been voted the "friendliest" in my high school class—but this well-meaning chatter was cutting into my research. For a while, I tried piling my canvas bags and overcoat on the adjacent seat as a signal that I preferred to be left alone. When the bus was full, however, the driver told me to use the overhead rack. As luck would have it, a neighborhood friend of mine with previous sales experience needed a job. I thought he might be able to work in Drexel's sales department. He could learn about the financial markets and we could commute together. He accepted my job offer and sat next to me on the bus in blessed silence.

When winter approached, the daylight hours grew short and I found it difficult to read under the flickering lights of the bus. So I purchased a medical headlamp—the kind surgeons strap to their heads—to improve the illumination. A bit unusual, perhaps, but it worked.

THE CUBE AND THE PYRAMID

Even before graduating from Wharton, I had been making presentations to Drexel's senior management. Describing my operations work in 1969, I had inserted several other concepts including the prosperity formula from my Berkeley days.

These ideas were part of my first financial speech in New York. It was called "The Best Investor Is a Social Scientist." By that, I meant you could know all about a company, but if you don't understand the social and regulatory trends acting on the company, you'd be less successful.

All this was wrapped together in a graphic labeled "The Corporate Financing Cube," a concept I had devised at Wharton. It showed that the best way to match a company's capital structure to its business risk was to account for six environmental factors: company, industry, capital markets, economy, regulation, and society.[*]

The next idea was what I called "the inverted pyramid" of Wall Street priorities. I had concluded that research could be the key to institutional competitive success on the Street. Most firms placed the greatest value on their sales staffs; next came trading; the research

---

[*] The fourth quarter 2002 edition of the *Milken Institute Review* contains a detailed explanation of the cube concept. See https://mikemilken.com/articles.taf?page=1.

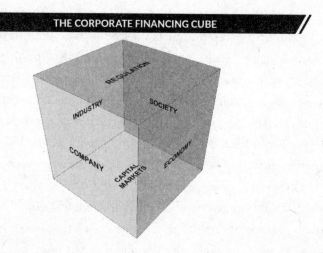

THE CORPORATE FINANCING CUBE

staff was underemphasized and undercompensated. I proposed to turn that upside down and make research our greatest competitive advantage.*

Over the next two years, I traveled the country talking to institutional customers about credit. Some of these companies had run into financial difficulty and needed help. It was similar to the intensive care a very sick hospital patient needs. Thus, I entered what I think of as my "clinical trials" period. It was a chance to prove my financial theories the same way a pharmaceutical company proves the efficacy of a new drug candidate.

The lower market value of many distressed companies created an opportunity for them to rebuild and recover by adjusting their capital structures with additional equity-linked securities. Companies we financed were able to save jobs by doing just that. I described this process in a series of research papers about various industries including defense contractors, airlines, railroads, and aerospace manufacturers.

---

* When I first became heavily involved in the search for medical solutions in the 1970s, I found a similar phenomenon: The most emphasis was placed on treatment, less on prevention, and very little on research. As in finance, I advocated inverting this pyramid so research would form the base of progress against diseases.

As the securities we wrote about rose in value, our firm burnished its already strong reputation as the leading research house. By 1972, I was no longer heading only research, but also running the entire fixed income department. Following a merger with Burnham and Company, I became head of the high yield and convertible bond department. The merged company agreed that all the department employees could keep 35 percent of any profits we earned after every expense, including salaries. Sixty-five percent went to the firm.

This percentage remained unchanged all the years I worked at Drexel, as did my salary, which had grown to $52,000.* Despite these broader responsibilities, I retained the view that we should base all our work on solid research. We dug deep to uncover hidden value and delivered strong results for the firm's clients. I contributed to this research by devoting my considerable commuting time to poring over company, industry, and regulatory reports.

STARTING THE MARATHON

One night, I arrived at our apartment just as Lori's mom was calling. She said she'd been treated for malignant breast cancer after her doctor discovered a lump during a routine screening. She was told it would be five years before she could be considered cured. At the time, I knew a lot about polio from research on my father's childhood affliction, but I knew little about cancer.

Lori and I were concerned her mom's condition could be life-threatening. It had been only a year since President Nixon famously declared "war on cancer." Unaware of any battles that had been won

---

* The percentage of profits retained by employees varied by department, with some receiving as much as 60 percent. But my department's split never changed from the original 35 percent. From time to time, other firms offered us substantially more to jump ship, but we never did.

in that war, I launched into a study of the disease—and of the infra-structure for treating it—in the hope I might find some information that would be useful in dealing with our family situation. Little did I know that my layman's study of cancer would be only the first mile of a decades-long marathon to accelerate cures for a wide range of serious diseases.*

The next mile in that marathon was another cancer scare in the family. One day in the early 1970s, my father noticed a sore on one of his big toes. He thought about getting it checked, but he was busy with clients and, in his mind, their needs always came first. Finally, at my mother's urging, he went to a doctor. A biopsy showed it was mel-anoma, a dangerous skin cancer, but the doctor assured him they'd caught it in time and the affected area could be removed safely. After researching the disease and the leading area surgeons, I returned to Los Angeles and took Dad to see a specialist, who reassured us about the prognosis.

THE BIRTH OF NEW FINANCIAL MARKETS

Convinced that these two cancer situations no longer needed urgent attention, I returned to work, where the department was growing fast. It eventually expanded to many divisions that provided a full range of services.

A decade later, some of our competitors, who were struggling to compete with the services we offered, started disparaging high-yield

---

* This was also the beginning of our philanthropy, which expanded over the next several years as our work produced more wealth. At first, Lori and I just wrote checks when we thought there was an opportunity to advance progress against cancer and other worthy causes. As our giving became more significant in the late 1970s, my brother and I made plans to formalize the charitable process by establishing foundations and hiring a profes-sional staff.

securities as "junk" and the media played along, forever associating me with what they liked to call "junk bonds." Yet the non-investment-grade debt business was only one of several divisions in the growing department.

A big challenge to my academic theories also came in 1974, the most important year in financial history since World War II. Throughout the early seventies, the trust banks promoted an investing strategy based on the "nifty fifty"—a group of large-capitalization stocks that had consistent earnings. Just buy and hold a basket of these stocks, the advice went, and you'd be successful. It was one-decision investing. For a while, the nifty fifty delivered on the promise.

To use a public health metaphor, the broad market had been healthy, with only limited outbreaks of weakness that were confined to a few industries or asset categories. But just as the COVID-19 pandemic followed earlier limited outbreaks like SARS and Ebola, a full financial pandemic was about to sweep global markets. It began with the OPEC oil embargo, Watergate, and stagflation. The Dow Jones Industrial Average fell 45 percent between January 1973 and December 1974, unemployment and inflation soared, interest rates shot up, and large financial institutions stopped lending to all but their highest-rated borrowers.

These changes led investors to look elsewhere for better returns and opened the way for rapid growth in the number and size of mutual funds. By providing alternative ways to finance business growth through debt obligations and other securities, the capital markets powered economic expansion into the 1980s and beyond.

That gave entrepreneurs greater access to growth capital. It was a change from "Whom do you know?" to "What can you do?" But in the mid-1970s, financial firms were suffering from a crisis of confidence. Many feared the dark days of 1929 were returning. Thousands of below-investment-grade and formerly investment-grade debt instruments were then tagged as junk because their issuers seemed on the verge of bankruptcy.

My advice to clients was to stay the course, look for value, and take advantage of opportunities—especially in beaten-down companies with high-quality management. Our research showed that the debt of many good companies could be bought for pennies on the dollar. Yes, there were severe strains on the financial system, but it seemed clear to me—based on solid data—that both the stock and bond markets were excessively oversold. Leading business publications ran stories questioning whether investors would ever again buy stocks.

The media were wrong. As the Dow neared bottom on December 6, 1974, it was a great opportunity to invest. Putting into practice everything I had studied and learned, I told clients our organization stood ready to help them.

Over the next two years, stocks and bonds recovered dramatically. A portfolio of non-investment-grade debt generated an unleveraged return of 100 percent. It was real-world proof of the academic theories I'd developed over the previous decade. Everything our organization had built in the six years since 1970—especially its emphasis on research—prevailed through a financial pandemic and established our credibility. That laid the foundation for the next stage in our growth so we could successfully finance thousands of companies that would create millions of jobs.

One by-product of this success was that by 1976 I had become independently wealthy. That fact alone was of little importance to me except that it created new career options. Having often returned to Wharton, where I happily engaged with the professors and their students, I considered becoming a full-time academic.

The chairman of our firm, I.W. Burnham, had close ties to Penn. When he heard rumors that I might leave Drexel, he invited me to lunch. "Mike," he said, "I understand the appeal of teaching and you'll always be able to do that part-time. But you're beginning to make a real impact on improving the financial system. Think about it." I realized that progress toward my career goals was just getting started. By staying in the for-profit financial arena, I'd be better able to expand capital access and build the industries of the future. Mr. Burnham agreed to help make that possible by increasing the amount of capital my team could manage.

Those first six years of the 1970s gave birth to new financial markets and new types of securities that stimulated economic growth and job creation, which continues today. Many other financial firms took part in this revolution following 1976. Starting in 1977, Drexel and others began expanding the original issuance of non-investment-grade securities. The growth of private equity—direct investment in unlisted companies that aligned the interests of management and ownership—also began in this period.

Today, the heads of many leading financial institutions who worked with me will say their businesses are modeled on the lessons of the 1970s and 1980s. There would be future financial crises caused by different factors: In the 1980s, it was overinvestment in sovereign debt and real estate; in 2008, an unsustainable residential housing bubble fueled by unwise use of leverage; and in 2020, a pandemic-caused jobs recession. But modern capital markets, whose solid foundation was established in the 1970s, have shown remarkable resilience in coping with these disruptions.

As America approached the two hundredth anniversary of the 1776 Declaration of Independence, I saw a bright, unlimited future. What I didn't realize was just how much my life was about to change.

FIVE

Every Parent's Fear

———

After our first child was born in May 1973, the apartment was getting crowded. Since we planned to have more children, we began looking for a place that would accommodate kids, visiting relatives, and out-of-town friends. The next year, we moved to a house in another Cherry Hill neighborhood. Our second son was born in December 1975. When he was about two months old, Lori's parents, Murray and Helen Hackel, came to visit and help out.

One night after dinner, I was clearing the table while Lori was in the nursery with the baby. Helen and Murray were in our two-year-old son's room getting him ready for bed. Suddenly, I heard loud anguished cries from Helen and ran up the short flight of stairs. Our boy was in Murray's arms shaking uncontrollably. Lori ran in holding the naked baby, saw what was happening, and screamed.

If you've never seen someone have a grand mal seizure—the violent spasms, the loss of consciousness—I assure you it's terrifying, even more so when the first one is your own child. Neither Lori nor I had seen one and we shared the same frightening thought: *Is our child dying?*

We called emergency services and raced to a nearby community hospital. Lori sat with our boy in the back of the ambulance while I followed in our car. Thinking back on those moments, it wasn't the safest situation—I was worried sick and drove too fast, the streets were dark, the roads were slick, and the siren wailed in my ears. It's all kind of a blur. Fortunately, Murray and Helen were able to stay behind and babysit.

After our son was admitted, the hospital staff said we couldn't stay in his room, so we tried to sleep as best we could on chairs in the waiting area. In such anguished times, you remember things that might otherwise have gone unnoticed: the medicinal smell of the hospital floor after the nightly mopping; beeping monitors; harsh fluorescent lights; muffled conversations between doctors and nurses down the hall. *Are they talking about our child?*

DR. CLIPBOARD

The next morning Lori and I were in our son's room when a doctor came in. He seemed uncaring, almost indifferent to his suffering patient. Without looking at Lori or me, he addressed his clipboard in an arrogant voice. "I've started him on ampicillin. It's probably spinal meningitis. To be sure, he needs to have a spinal tap. Fill out this authorization form and someone will be in to take him for the procedure."

As I started to read the form, Lori stood on her toes hoping she could lean over far enough to kiss our son. His eyes were closed and we couldn't tell if he was sleeping or not.

Once we signed the papers, a nurse wheeled the crib to a procedure room on the other side of the hospital. We knew our frightened little boy woke up because even at a distance, we heard him shrieking in pain as they inserted a large needle in his back. Each of his cries was like a knife in my side.

Over the next few days, our firstborn suffered more than anyone should have to endure. Even more than the pain, we were so worried about how terrified he must have been.

The doctor in charge of his case said he most likely had experienced a febrile seizure, which is fairly common in young children. Given a high-enough temperature, everyone will have a seizure, although some have a lower trigger point than others. It's part of the body's protective mechanism. Common or not, we weren't getting clear answers about why he was so sick.

I began researching all the possible causes of seizures, a scary list of conditions that included fatal brain tumors. I started calling other doctors I knew around the country looking for information.

We took turns at the hospital, alternating between sitting at our little boy's bedside to comfort him, bringing him toys, interrogating the doctors, and succumbing to periods of fitful sleep in the waiting room. On the second day, Helen joined us, but since only two visitors were allowed in the room, she waited in the hall.

We'd heard that one sign of meningitis is a stiff neck. Lori asked our boy if he could move his neck, but he just stared at us and said "No, it hurts." I walked to the other side of the crib, raised my hand with two fingers up, and asked him to tell me how many fingers he saw. He would have to turn his head to see them. No answer. Eyes staring up at nothing.

Then "Dr. Clipboard" returned, giving his little patient only a cursory glance: "The spinal tap results were inconclusive," he began. "We have to repeat it because he's not responding the way he should." Lori burst into tears and hurried out to the hall. "He'll be fine," her mother assured her. "He comes from strong stock." That was said with the same defiance and determination of her Russian forbears who'd escaped the pogroms to cross the Atlantic—first to Ellis Island, then Chicago and San Francisco before settling permanently in Los Angeles.

The third day, we brought our little patient a present, a Fisher-Price cash register. His eyes followed the cash register from Lori's hands into the crib, then stopped, staring at it. He didn't move. I leaned over the crib and pushed the buttons on the cash register to make it ring. "Want to try it?" Just then Lori said, "Stop the ringing. Look at his neck. Does it look red to you?"

When the doctor came in, Lori pointed out the redness. He looked down at our son, as if afraid to touch him, and used his index finger to push the hospital gown aside. A red rash was spreading like strawberry jam over his chest. "It's an allergic reaction to the ampicillin," he said casually as if it was a splinter instead of the life-threatening danger it could have become had it not been detected. Scribbling on his clipboard, the doctor said, "I'll have his antibiotic switched. He needs another spinal tap."

Lori and I had discussed that possibility and I said, "We really don't want to put him through another one." For the first time, the doctor looked up: "Then take him and get out! He can't stay here if you refuse treatment." We signed the form.

The following day when we arrived, our son was standing in the crib. We were thrilled when he greeted us with a loud "Where's my present?"

By day four, he seemed much better, although we still lacked a definitive diagnosis. After a few more days, we brought him home with discharge instructions on how to respond if he had another seizure.

The final diagnosis was not spinal meningitis, but a febrile seizure. When we told Lori's parents, Helen informed us that she had had seizures as a child, as did Lori and her sister. They'd outgrown them and she was sure our son would also. (At the time, genetic testing was not available. It wasn't until many years later that Dr. Pete Engel—an expert whose work at UCLA we funded—discovered a relevant gene. Now, with genetic testing and family histories, we've traced the condition through five generations.)

I intensified my study of both his condition and the leading pediatric medical facilities. It turned out that Children's Hospital of Philadelphia (CHOP), only a few miles across the Delaware River, had long been ranked the best children's hospital in the United States. CHOP had recently built a new hospital adjacent to the University of Pennsylvania Medical Center. When our son had a third grand mal seizure after a few more weeks, we took him straight to CHOP.

After extensive tests, the Children's Hospital doctors diagnosed him with a specific form of epilepsy that can begin with febrile seizures. That lifted a heavy cloud of uncertainty—it was a relief to have a clear diagnosis. The condition was serious, but it was treatable. My fear about a brain tumor faded. Armed with a diagnosis, I dug deeper for information, consulting several major drug companies and visiting the National Institute of Neurological Disorders and Stroke (NINDS) in Bethesda, Maryland. This search became a new branch of my career path.

In many cases, epilepsy is never controlled. It can recur after uneventful years, even decades. When seizures are limited to infancy, a child may grow up without realizing they happened. But a parent can never forget. Never. It's burned into our memories. I will always remember that first episode. It tears your heart out to see a small child's eyes roll back in his or her head when they lose consciousness. You feel so helpless, not only during the active phase of the convulsions, but also later when it can be difficult to wake a child up or bring him out of his confused state.

FRIGHTENED KIDS, ANXIOUS PARENTS

As concerned as we were about our son, we realized that other parents must deal with even more serious conditions, and often with fewer resources to handle the situation. One day in the waiting area at CHOP, Lori and I met the woman whose daughter shared our son's room. The little girl had already endured two heart operations. Now she faced a third surgery because she was starting to turn blue. You can imagine the mother's anxiety, made worse by the fact that they had no savings and her husband couldn't afford to take more than one day off from his hourly job. What an overwhelming dilemma—having to be at work and not knowing the results of the surgery that determines whether your child will live or die.

Other parents stay at hospitals for emotionally draining weeks while their children undergo extended treatments. Many come to specialized hospitals from distant cities and don't have the options we had. They can't put their jobs on hold. Some of those who are able to stay nearby can't afford the lodging costs. On top of medical bills and travel expenses, they have to pay for care of other children left at home.

Lori and I were early supporters of such organizations as the Ronald McDonald House Charities, which had been founded in Philadelphia in 1974, two years before our first experience with a seizure. This wonderful philanthropy provides a home away from home that gives comfort and resources to families who must travel for their children's medical care. A few years later, when my brother and I created the Milken Family Foundation, we focused on social programs for families whose children were undergoing treatment.

Parents never stop worrying. The images of a medical time bomb are always in your mind. *What if he has a seizure in a swimming pool or climbing on a jungle gym?* Later, when she gets a driver's license: *Is it safe to let her get behind the wheel? Can she safely bear children?* Seizures can return at any point throughout life. Tragedies can happen to anyone, anywhere: John Travolta's son died when his head hit the edge of a bathtub during a seizure.

All three of our children have suffered from epileptic seizures, as have some of our grandchildren. I remember holding our little girl in my arms when she suddenly started shaking; her oldest brother had been seizure-free for more than a decade when he collapsed in spasms while running during a high school cross-country event. We've been fortunate that advanced therapies have controlled their seizures so they've been able to enjoy full, productive lives. We established the Milken Family Foundation Epilepsy Research Awards program in association with the American Epilepsy Society to accelerate neuroscience research that can improve the outcomes of people with all forms of the condition.

A key advisor on our epilepsy awards was Dr. W. Donald Shields, head of pediatric neurology at UCLA for more than a quarter century. Don has been a great medical resource and friend to our family since the early 1980s. Don grew up in Utah—his great-great-grandfather was Brigham Young, the religious leader, founder of Salt Lake City, and first governor of the Utah Territory.

Recipients of our Early Career Physician-Scientist Awards and our Translational Research Awards have greatly advanced the science of epilepsy diagnosis and treatment. Neuroimaging and neurogenetics have transformed how doctors plan therapeutic strategies. The number of available anti-seizure drugs has doubled, reducing unwanted adverse effects and providing greater choices for individual patients. Surgical therapy has also improved so that many more patients are eligible for surgery. New techniques like focused ultrasound, laser ablation, and neuromodulation have provided relief for patients who are not candidates for standard surgery. Finally, many more developing countries with limited resources now have specialized epilepsy centers. Still, there's much to do before parents of epileptic children can relax.

When Lori and I first learned about epilepsy forty-seven years ago, it set us on a new course, a quest that has never let up. Back in 1976, we began to understand that all parents share a bond. We speak to other parents often about neurology research that offers greater hope for all kids at risk.

SIX

Life Gets in the Way

Winston Churchill once observed that if everyone knew the future, the present would be intolerable. For better or worse, life is full of surprises. It happens, as John Lennon sang, when you're busy making other plans.

By the summer of 1976, medication had suppressed our son's seizures. That August, Lori and I planned a trip to California to see our families and friends. We stayed with Lori's parents because they had two extra bedrooms for the four of us. It wasn't far from my parents' house where there was less space because my younger sister still lived there.

When I visited my parents the next day, it struck me that Dad looked tired and, well, older. His bout with melanoma a few years earlier had been treated as a localized condition. There's always a risk of metastasis with melanoma, but it hadn't seemed life-threatening at the time. Nevertheless, that was when I first brought him to

Dr. Donald Morton, a well-known Los Angeles specialist who was working to develop a vaccine therapy for skin cancers. It was the beginning of what is now nearly five decades of supporting melanoma research. Over the next few years between 1974 and 1976, I'd developed a strong relationship with Don and learned much about the disease through my interactions with the National Cancer Institute and major medical centers. I knew that if a localized melanoma reoccurred in a distant organ, the outlook was very poor.

Dad told me he'd recently seen Dr. Morton and his cancer had returned. It was far worse this time. Cancer cells were no longer confined to his toe—they were spreading through his body.

I felt a chill despite the August heat. The same feeling—tightness in my chest, a lump in my stomach—that hit me only months earlier when our son was hospitalized was overcoming me again. Thoughts raced through my mind. It had been four years since my mother-in-law's breast cancer diagnosis and she was doing well—her doctor said she was cancer-free. Dad's condition seemed to be different. I hadn't yet figured out the best way to proceed. What I knew for sure, however, was that I wouldn't be able to tell him all the things I'd been planning to say about my work. None of that mattered now—*Dad needs my help.*

One irony is that he never had the chance to tell *his* father about his success—how he had put himself through college and law school, built a thriving accounting practice, raised a happy family, and become an admired community leader. All that happened after his father, my grandfather, died in an auto accident.

DEFINITION OF A REAL PROBLEM

I immediately scheduled another appointment for Dad to see Dr. Morton. Don was an esteemed doctor and a remarkable man. The son of a West Virginia coal miner, he rose through the medical ranks to become head of surgical oncology at UCLA. Later, he developed a groundbreaking diagnostic technique—the sentinel lymph node biopsy—that has spared millions of patients from unnecessary and disfiguring operations. Eventually, he moved to the Saint John's Health Center in Santa Monica, where he founded the John Wayne Cancer Institute, named after the famous actor, whom he had treated.

Although Don was a large bear of a man, he was never intimidating. After examining Dad again and reviewing the medical record, he was kind, but realistic. Melanoma, he explained, is one of the fastest-growing cancers. A billion cells in January could become a trillion cells by December. And it was too early to tell if his vaccine would work. At the time, metastatic melanoma was almost universally fatal. (Today, thanks to research breakthroughs sponsored by the Melanoma Research Alliance, under the auspices of the Milken Institute, patients have much better prognoses.)

Despite the pessimistic outlook, I wasn't ready to give up. There must be a solution. *I can't just sit back and let him die!* If we consult enough specialists, pursue every medical option, the answer has to be there . . . somewhere. There had never been a serious problem I couldn't solve—I could refinance any company, overcome any financial issue. Surely the solution would be within my grasp.

In addition to UCLA, we visited major medical centers around the country including Johns Hopkins in Baltimore, MD Anderson Cancer Center in Houston, Penn Medicine in Philadelphia, the Dana-Farber Cancer Institute in Boston, and the Sloan-Kettering Institute (now Memorial Sloan Kettering Cancer Center) in New York. But the state of the science just hadn't progressed enough. After several months, I came to an anguished and depressing conclusion: The definition of a real problem is something that can't be solved with money. It was a crushing realization that my father might die. Never, before or since, have I been so overcome by a feeling of emptiness. I had to accept the probability that nothing anyone did could accelerate science enough to save him. Still, I held on to a shred of hope until very near the end of his life.

Forty-seven years later, as I reflect on the years before and after 1976, it becomes clear that that annus horribilis was the fulcrum of my life. I felt I'd achieved great success in my financial career and was just starting on the quest to advance medical solutions. After 1976, the search for faster cures became a second focus. Now I had two careers of equal importance. It started with a few diseases—melanoma, breast cancer, epilepsy—and then, when we'd created the template, all potentially fatal conditions.

MOVING WEST

Lori and I began planning a permanent move back to California. With two young boys, we had moved from our Cherry Hill, New Jersey, apartment to a house. Now we'd move again. I wanted our two boys to know their grandfather in the time he had left; and I wanted him to know them. It took some time to negotiate the transfer of my department at Drexel from New York to California. I told the firm I'd understand if they couldn't accept my request to move.

Once details were settled, I announced the news at our department's 1976 holiday party. Not everyone in my group was in favor of the plan. (The following year, one colleague told me I should see the new Woody Allen movie *Annie Hall*, which made fun of the California lifestyle.) But we tried to make the transition as easy as possible for the affected employees by helping them find housing, schools, and jobs for spouses. Every employee of the department had an opportunity to visit California and was free to stay in New York or move with us. Either way, their jobs were secure. Ninety-three percent of them chose to join me. The other 7 percent had important personal obligations that precluded a move.

Before buying a house in 1977, Lori and I explored several areas and concluded we wanted to live in a diverse middle-class neighborhood. One requirement was a nearby hospital given the kids' medical issues. We also wanted them to be able to walk to school. California public schools—Hesby Street, Birmingham, and Berkeley—had given us a fine education and I assumed that most relocating employees would send their kids to Los Angeles public institutions. We finally moved in 1978 and after we enrolled our older boy, we were shocked to learn that he was the only one in the neighborhood attending public school. It wasn't just our neighborhood—almost all the relocated employees sent their children to private schools. I hadn't appreciated just how much primary and secondary education in Los Angeles had changed.

Along with my brother, Lowell, we vowed to do something about it.* Soon we began planning to establish private foundations that could provide professional structure for our previous individual philanthropy. These groups, which were planned in the late 1970s and formally launched in early 1982, were eventually consolidated into what is today the Milken Family Foundation. (I can't tell you how many hundreds of inaccurate media stories continue to report that I "turned to" philanthropy much later, in the 1990s.)

---

* Lowell Milken is widely recognized as one of the most thoughtful and effective leaders in the field of education. His groundbreaking initiatives reflect a core commitment to education as essential to America's future leadership, prosperity, and security.

TREASURING EVERY DAY

Because I was so busy building my department and arranging to move the business across the country, it was difficult to get back to Los Angeles as often as I wanted. I called my father regularly to see how he was doing. While Dad was still able to travel, I arranged for him and my mother to visit us. It's funny how you remember a particular day half a century later. I have this vivid memory of him sitting on the floor playing with our two sons in the basement of our New Jersey house.

Although Dad never knew the extent of my financial success, Lori and I were able to provide a European vacation for the entire family—my parents, Lori's parents, my brother and his wife, Lori's sister and her husband, Lori and I. Dad questioned whether I could afford such a long trip. I told him not to worry. None of them had been to Europe except for Lori's father, and he had not been back since the D-Day invasion more than thirty years earlier.

We arrived permanently in Los Angeles just before my thirty-second birthday on the Fourth of July, 1978. Soon we moved into the new house where we would raise our three kids—our daughter was born in 1980—and where Lori and I still live. Dad survived nine and a half months after we moved. Although he was declining, he got to be a grandpa with his grandsons close by.

During this time, there'd been an old weeping willow tree in the front yard of our house. The tree was sick, too, under attack by a fungus, and I began to see it as a symbol of my father. Keeping this tree alive became my mission. Seemingly, every tree expert in Southern California came to treat it. I'd done the equivalent for my dad, of course, but now there appeared to be no path forward for him. The tree had more time. He did not.

Lori read me her diary entry from March 24, 1979, one of our last visits with Dad. We attempted to play bridge, but he was too weak. His face looked skeletal and his mind was dulled by pain pills. Playing bridge was beyond him that night, or any night to come. Lori's diary says "Bernard died tonight." He didn't actually pass away until April 18, Lori's birthday, but I knew what she meant. The active, happy father who had been my guide and inspiration was no longer there.

The tree in our yard survived and went on living for a few years. Trees, of course, are not people. We live on different timescales. But it struck me then that science was moving at a slow pace more appropriate to the life span of some trees, not humans. Cures weren't coming fast enough. I needed to figure out how we could pick up the pace, especially since my father was only one of many relatives and friends stricken by deadly diseases.

*   *   *

DISEASE AS A MOTIVATOR

Several months before my father died, I had been in Palm Springs—what we Californians call "the desert"—for a charity event. The local tourist guides say midwinter is a perfect time for pool lounging and spa pampering. I was never into those activities, but do enjoy walking in the warm, dry air. It was the first time I'd been there since my parents took me as a kid. One of my two first cousins, Stanley Gore, was visiting with his wife, Barbara, and we decided to go for a walk.

Stanley was a lawyer in his midthirties—a few years older than I—and appeared to be in fine health. We walked briskly in the shadow of the San Jacinto Mountains. The next time I saw Stanley was at my father's funeral. On that sorrowful occasion, he mentioned he'd been having headaches and sometimes his vision was blurred. I suggested he get checked by a neurologist. A month later, we learned he'd been diagnosed with a tumor on his brain stem.

The prognosis for Stanley was grim, but I immediately called Dr. Neal Kassell, a leading neurosurgeon then at the University of Virginia. Neal and I had met ten years earlier when he was a medical student at the University of Pennsylvania and I was at Penn's Wharton School, a few blocks away. He planned to launch a medical start-up company and needed financing. One of my Wharton professors told him I might provide some advice.

Over the years, Neal and I spoke frequently. I'd reached out to him when my son had his first seizures and later when my stepfather had glioblastoma. On this occasion, Neal reviewed the state of brain cancer science and offered to refer Stanley to some nearby specialists. But he was realistic about the vanishingly small possibility of a cure. A few months later, Lori and I attended Stanley's funeral.

With all the progress we've made—today many cancers are manageable—we sometimes forget how the very word "cancer" used to strike terror into all patients. In 1971, the beginning of what President Nixon called the "War on Cancer," most people considered it a death sentence. When I interviewed President George W. Bush at the Milken Institute Global Conference a few years ago, he told the story of his sister, Robin, who died from leukemia in 1953 before her fourth birthday. Robin's father, President George H. W. Bush, was one of twenty-two American presidents who'd lost a child. Clearly, disease has no respect for wealth or high public office.

CHANGING THE PROCESS

The impact of diseases on my family—my father, mother-in-law, children, cousins, and others—was becoming overwhelming. What,

I asked myself, could accelerate medical science and change history? I had to figure something out. It would require far more than my childhood study of polio, the cause of my father's limp; more than I'd learned about breast cancer after my mother-in-law's diagnosis. Real change would require a deeper understanding of the medical research *process*.

In 1982, the first in a series of our private foundations began making grants to support innovations in education and health. We also established medical research awards programs that provided individual grants up to $250,000.

Those who received awards in the 1980s included Dr. Dennis Slamon, who discovered Herceptin, a revolutionary breakthrough in the treatment of one type of breast cancer; Dr. Bert Vogelstein, who did pioneering work on the incalculably important p53 gene whose mutant form is believed to be involved in more than half of human cancers; Dr. Lawrence Einhorn, who devised a platinum-based chemotherapy regimen that cures testicular cancers;* Dr. Philip Leder, a pioneer in molecular biology who contributed to the deciphering of the genetic code; Dr. Ernst Wynder, credited with coauthoring the first study definitively linking lung cancer and smoking; and many more.

In our search for solutions, we made philanthropic gifts to hundreds of worthwhile causes. No doubt these did some good, but I couldn't shake the feeling we weren't really speeding up medical science.

---

* I thought about Dr. Einhorn when Joe Torre, then the manager of the New York Yankees, called me one day about twenty years ago. Joe asked me to speak to a young man diagnosed with testicular cancer who had declined to undergo treatment because he feared terrible side effects. I explained to this patient that his cancer used to have only a 5 percent long-term survival rate. Now, thanks to new protocols, the success rate is more than 95 percent. We spoke by phone several times. When he understood that a few months of treatment offered him the prospect of a long healthy life, he agreed it was worth it to begin the therapy.

Meanwhile, in 1980, we created a medical concierge service for any employee, relative, friend, or even a client facing a life-threatening disease. We developed substantial expertise in finding the best doctors and hospitals to meet their needs. That tradition continues in all our organizations today.

THE LIST IS LONG

Over the years, many more close relatives succumbed to serious or fatal illnesses and accidents. Beyond our family, the list of ill-fated friends and associates is long. Some, like Magic Johnson and Joe Torre, are well-known sports figures and, thankfully, continue to lead full lives after dealing with life-threatening diseases. Others, like economist Gary Becker; *Wall Street Journal* editor Bob Bartley; AIDS activist Elizabeth Glaser; and Memorial Sloan Kettering urology chief Dr. Bill Fair, were simply among the best in their fields before they succumbed.

In some cases, I never had an opportunity to say good-bye to good friends. One of these was Reginald Lewis, who came from a tough East Baltimore neighborhood and through sheer grit became a star athlete, a Harvard-trained lawyer, and a remarkably successful entrepreneur. During the 1980s, my firm and others helped finance the growth of the business that made Reg one of the first African Americans to lead a billion-dollar enterprise. I called him the Jackie Robinson of business. His success bookended my quest—begun in Watts two decades earlier—to expand access to capital for minorities.

He personified what the marriage of capital and ability could achieve when financing decisions as color-blind as possible. Reg analyzed opportunities skillfully, conducted thorough due diligence, and handled the deals. We formed a close bond and toured the country to inspire minority students with the message that any one of them could be the next great entrepreneur.

Reg came to see me one day in 1992 and asked how he could contact Neal Kassell, the neurosurgeon who had been my good friend since graduate school. Reg and Neal had met briefly at one of our cancer awards dinners. I should have made the connection, but only in retrospect did I realize that Reg's visit was to say good-bye to me. I didn't know—no one knew—that at the height of his career, he had been diagnosed with a glioblastoma and had refused all treatment. He preferred to let the brain tumor take him fast rather than fight it and linger in a weakened body. Until almost the end, he told no one he was sick. Reg left instructions that he was to be buried with his tennis racket and a bottle of Dom Pérignon.

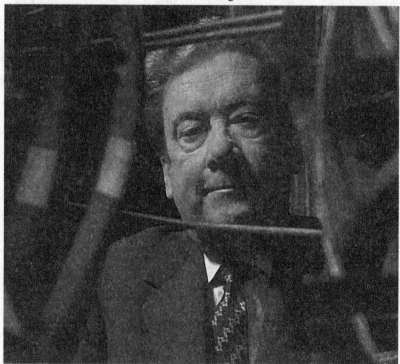

Bill McGowan.

His game was tennis, but to use a golf metaphor, how sad he never had a chance to play the back nine.

DRIVEN TO FOCUS

William McGowan was one of America's great business leaders. His tiny company, MCI, took on AT&T, the industry colossus with a 98 percent market share, and succeeded in creating the world's first fiber-optic network, the backbone of today's internet. When I met Bill in the late 1970s, he was spending most of his time trying to raise capital. Eventually, we raised $2.6 billion for MCI, freeing Bill to run his successful business. The only thing that could stop him was heart disease, which led to two heart attacks, a heart transplant, and his death in 1992 before I could see him one last time.

And then there's Steven Ross, the larger-than-life chairman of Time Warner, who had remarkable gifts for leadership, finance, and technology. He also may have had one of the unhealthiest diets, a fact that may have contributed to his prostate cancer. I've always believed that Time Warner would have become a very different company if Steve had lived longer. He was on my mind when, at age forty-six, I asked a doctor for a prostate-specific antigen test that led to my own cancer diagnosis.

Reg Lewis, Bill McGowan, and Steve Ross died within months of each other in 1992 and 1993. Each was far more than a client. They are just a few of the friends, family, and associates whose struggles with disease motivated my search for cures. Unfortunately, the full list of those who have suffered is much longer. That's why I'm constantly driven to focus on the science as the best way to accelerate progress. In doing that, my guide is the same principle I've applied in business—empower the most talented people in each field and encourage them to pursue their passions.

PART II

No Longer Just a Donor

SEVEN

"You Have Cancer"

The internist who examined me did the usual poking and prodding of a routine physical exam. Then I asked for a simple blood test for prostate cancer. "You're only forty-six," he said. "That's too young. Maybe in five or ten years." But I persisted, in part because my friend Steve Ross, the late chairman of Time Warner, had passed away from that disease on December 20, 1992, just a month earlier.

The doctor called me in a few days. "Good news," he began in a cheerful tone. "Your cholesterol is fine and everything else looks good. There's just one thing and I'm sure it's a lab mistake. Your prostate-specific antigen blood test—PSA—looks a bit high on this printout. It says twenty-four but, as I said, it's probably a mistake. Just to be sure, we should check it again. In the meantime, don't worry about it."

Some quick research told me that the upper limit of the normal

PSA range is four nanograms per milliliter. If mine really was twenty-four, six times the upper limit of normal, there was reason for concern. Yet even a reading that high doesn't necessarily mean cancer. There are other causes of a high PSA, including an infection, inflammation, and a larger-than-usual prostate gland. If those causes are ruled out and a second blood test shows the same result, the next step would be a biopsy to look for cancer cells.

While I waited for further test results, there was time to conduct more research. Foremost in my mind were patients who had failed to take aggressive action at the first sign of what could be cancer. Over the years, it had become clear to me that many people do too little at the beginning of their clinical odysseys, and then—when the disease burden is greater—will do anything to survive.

SPREADING THE NET

Since the 1970s, I'd been supporting medical research and helping sick friends and relatives. Now I was the patient, possibly a cancer patient. The first step was to call several specialists at leading medical institutions like Memorial Sloan Kettering Cancer Center in New York, the Johns Hopkins University in Baltimore, the MD Anderson Cancer Center in Houston, and the National Cancer Institute outside Washington, DC. At the NCI, I quickly connected with Sam Broder, then the agency's director, and Steve Rosenberg, the very first participant in our young investigator program.

Some of these specialists had been recognized years earlier as winners of the Milken Family Foundation Cancer Research Awards. Through our work at the Foundation, I knew Patrick Walsh, the head of the clinical faculty at the Johns Hopkins Brady Urological

Institute.* At this point, it wasn't yet clear that I had cancer. Still, I thought, if I did have a cancerous prostate, I'd want to consult a good surgeon and Pat was one of the best. He was on the other side of the country in Baltimore and I'd probably need a local surgeon, but at least Pat might offer useful advice. He said he'd be glad to see me if further tests indicated that surgery was an option.

Next, I called Merv Adelson, a close friend whose prostate cancer had been treated successfully with surgery. Merv had cofounded Lorimar Television, which my firm financed for several years. They produced many hit TV shows including *Dallas*, *The Waltons*, *Knots Landing*, and *Falcon Crest*. (Later, Warner Communications, led by Steve Ross, purchased Lorimar.)

Merv strongly recommended his surgeon, Dr. Stuart "Skip" Holden, a specialist in urological oncology at Cedars-Sinai Medical Center in Los Angeles. I called Holden, who returned my call promptly, explaining he was between flights in the Atlanta airport on his way back to LA after a family event in Florida. He agreed to see me the next day. In the meantime, I collected every possible book and article about prostate cancer, and started taking notes. One article said 240,000 American men would be diagnosed with prostate cancer that year.

Hmmm, if it is cancer, I'm not exactly in a select group.

The next paragraph caught me up short: thirty-five thousand of these men would die and the estimates of future deaths were far worse. Because of an aging population, epidemiologists projected as

---

* Walsh is the author of *Dr. Patrick Walsh's Guide to Surviving Prostate Cancer*. Before his innovations, removal of a cancerous prostate meant the patient could become incontinent and impotent. Pat invented a procedure that spared the nerves surrounding the prostate, greatly improving most patients' quality of life by preserving sexual function and urinary control.

many as 150,000 annual deaths within two decades. Of course, that assumed no progress toward improved treatments and cures.

More than twenty years of involvement with medical researchers taught me a lot about many types of cancer and other serious diseases. But I didn't know enough yet about the prostate, the walnut-sized gland that harbors cancer in about one of every eight men.* About one in six African American men will be diagnosed with the disease.

That same day, I called my old friend Neal Kassell, the University of Virginia neurosurgeon I'd kept in touch with since we first met at Penn almost a quarter century earlier. He's treated many famous patients, including President Joe Biden when was still a senator. Neal wasn't a prostate expert, but I trusted his clinical instincts and appreciated his frankness. If anyone would tell me the unvarnished truth, he would.

Neal sometimes joked about the time he invited me to Penn medical school's anatomy lab to observe his dissection skills. When he cut into a monkey's brain, I almost fainted. My joking way of getting back at him for that caper was to threaten to make him sit through a lecture about the mathematical modeling of financial assets. In one sense, we had little in common—his studies of human brain structures and my studies of corporate capital structures occupied completely separate realms. But we became good friends, recognizing in each other a shared concern for helping people.

This time, I wasn't joking. "Neal, if you had prostate cancer, what's

---

* Each year, the American Cancer Society estimates the overall incidence of prostate cancer—the occurrence of new cases in the population. While I'm happy to report that the *death rate* from this disease has declined sharply (about 52 percent since 1993) because of improved treatments, the *incidence* did not change much. Yet the reported number has varied from one in five to one in nine. I don't believe fewer cases are occurring; in fact, there are probably more cases as our population ages. Rather, the reported variance may reflect two things: fewer men being tested because of what I consider an ill-advised recommendation of the US Preventive Services Task Force; and the reluctance of some doctors to label early disease as "cancer" so as not to alarm their patients.

the first thing you'd do?" He didn't miss a beat: "I'd call Andy von Eschenbach. He's the best. Do you want me to introduce you?"

Andrew von Eschenbach, MD, had known Neal from their days as surgical residents at Penn. Now he was the chair of urology at the University of Texas MD Anderson Cancer Center, one of the two or three top-rated cancer centers in the world.* (President George W. Bush later named Andy the director of the National Cancer Institute and then commissioner of the Food and Drug Administration.)

Andy and I spoke later that day and soon found we had much in common: Both of us were close to our fathers, who'd had a profound influence on our lives. Both of our fathers were diagnosed with cancer in the early 1970s. In the mid-1970s, Andy and I both learned that our fathers' cancers had spread, leaving a poor prognosis. We each took our fathers to distant cancer centers in search of a better outcome. They both died at the end of the 1970s leading each of us to rededicate ourselves to a search for medical solutions.

"I'll be happy to see you," Andy told me, "but it's kind of crazy around here right now because we're preparing to host a conference of prostate cancer specialists next week." When I said I'd like to attend this meeting, Andy was startled. He explained that only medical professionals would attend, not patients; but he agreed to let me in when I said I'd bring my urologist.

Things were moving fast. It had been less than forty-eight hours since the first call about my elevated PSA reading. Soon I was in Skip Holden's office looking for some reassurance that whatever this was, it could be quickly resolved. Years later, Holden recalled doing another PSA blood test and performing a digital rectal exam.

---

* More than fifteen years earlier, I had taken my father to MD Anderson, one of several centers where we sought advice and treatment for the malignant melanoma that eventually took his life.

As soon as I felt his prostate, I knew instantly that he had cancer and that it had spread. After decades of practicing urology, you can tell just by the condition of the prostate even before it's confirmed by a biopsy. This was not some subtle indication; it was very obvious. Another thing experience teaches you: Don't blurt out something like "Oh my God!" You keep your cool.

The next step was a needle biopsy. Dr. Holden extracted several cores of tissue from different areas of my prostate. One evaluation of the biopsy cores—called the Gleason score—measures a cancer's aggressiveness.* The results were bad—very bad. The pathologist's report said my cancer was in the "most aggressive" category. I never went back to that first doctor, the one who had been reluctant to test for cancer. I still shudder at the thought of what would have happened if I hadn't insisted on the PSA test even though I felt fine.

LET'S PREPARE FOR SURGERY

Skip says the most difficult part of his work is confirming the worst fears of worried patients that they have cancer. At first, I was devastated when he told me the bad news. But this was no time to be passive. Now that we knew it was cancer, my first thought was to get to the operating room and get rid of the thing. Unfortunately, the de-

---

* Looking at cancer cells under a microscope, pathologists assign two scores, each on a scale of one (normal) to five (most aggressive). The first number is given to the most predominant pattern of cell shape—how much they deviate from the shape of normal cells—and the second to the next-most-predominant pattern. The Gleason score (named for Dr. Donald Gleason, who developed it in the 1960s) is the sum of the two numbers. The highest (worst) score is ten. Every one of my cores scored in the nine to ten range. For more details, search "Gleason score" at pcf.org.

cision wasn't that simple. Imaging tests and another biopsy showed cancer had spread to my lymph nodes, which were grossly enlarged—some were swollen to dozens of times their normal size. That eliminates surgery as an option in most cases because once cancer escapes the prostate and spreads, doctors usually recommend against it. At that point, we didn't know if the cancer had spread beyond my lymph nodes. Given my high Gleason score, that was a possibility.

What now? Maybe get another opinion, this time from Dr. Jean DeKernion, the chief of urological oncology at UCLA, one of the nation's leading research institutions. DeKernion had a very distinguished résumé; no doubt he'd be able to reassure me that some definitive treatment would take care of this problem. He was well aware of our past support of many doctors at UCLA as they carried forward advanced, often miraculous, treatments for melanoma, breast cancer, childhood neurological disorders, and more. I had faith in them and in the process. So far, all the news about my situation had been negative, but I remained optimistic that he would offer an effective solution.

WHOA!

Lori joined me to meet with Dr. DeKernion at his UCLA office. As he studied my medical records and test results, I noted the wall behind him filled with framed diplomas, awards, and photos. Grateful patients would later endow a departmental chair in his honor. Lori sat on my left, pen in hand, ready to take notes about what we expected would be a discussion of various treatment options.

We discussed my case at length. He repeated what we already knew—that I had aggressive prostate cancer, that it had spread, and that surgery was not an alternative. As we spoke, I was thinking that at the very worst, I could look forward to some more healthy years.

My father had melanoma, one of the fastest-growing cancers, and he lived more than five years after his diagnosis. My mother-in-law survived twelve years with breast cancer before she succumbed to multiple myeloma. Confident we could attack this thing harder than they had, wouldn't my prognosis be better? So I asked the eminent Dr. DeKernion what he would do in my situation.

> *Mike, you can begin a course of androgen-deprivation therapy—hormones—that in about 90 percent of cases reduce the tumors. Then you have the option of radiation, which can buy you some more time. But you must understand that these treatments aren't a cure. Eventually, the cancer returns and there's nothing really effective over the long term.*
>
> *So here's my recommendation: First, get your affairs in order. Second, you and Lori should speak to a psychiatrist to help you deal with your terminal illness. And third, get a psychologist for your children to prepare them for what's coming.*

"Whoa! One thing at a time. I appreciate your recommendation," I said, "but there's a lot to think about, a lot to do, before considering getting my affairs in order. I'm not a patient who's ready to give up. We haven't even begun to fight this thing." Lori reached over and squeezed my hand. My first thoughts were about more than a dozen friends and relatives who had succumbed to various forms of cancer. But almost all of them were older at the time of diagnosis. *What could I do that they hadn't done? Am I going to see my kids graduate from college, get married, have kids of their own?*

My head was spinning. *Focus. Think. Plan. Work the plan. You know how. Just do it.*

That evening, Lori and I sat in bed and tried to make sense of all this new information. We discussed telling the kids about my cancer, but I said I wanted to wait until after the MD Anderson conference before telling the kids about my diagnosis. The explanation would be simple: I have cancer, but it will be treated and I'll be fine. We had a good cry and hugged each other for a very long time. Neither of us slept that night.

BOTTOMLESS PIT

Early the next morning, I called Skip Holden about Andy von Eschenbach's conference at MD Anderson. "It's funny you should call me about that conference, Mike. I'm sitting here looking at the conference brochure." We agreed that Skip and I would fly to Houston, where Andy would run some additional tests on me before hosting his event.

The weekend before that trip was an opportunity for more research. Among my many calls, one was to Dr. Charles "Snuffy" Myers, a medical oncologist and prostate cancer specialist I'd known for several years since he received one of our cancer research awards. Snuffy, who likes to say he works on both sides of the test tube—as a researcher and a clinician—was also planning to attend the Houston conference. He not only agreed to meet with me there, but also suggested we assemble a panel of specialists to review my case.

Another call went to Dr. Howard Scher at Memorial Sloan Kettering Cancer Center in New York. I told him that cancer had spread to my lymph nodes and Dr. DeKernion advised hormone treatment. Howard suggested we delay that treatment, which can cause mutations in the cancer cells. If I could come to his clinic for a needle biopsy of the lymph nodes, his team would then inject my cancer into some mice so they could test different therapies on the mice. We scheduled an appointment as soon as possible after the upcoming Houston trip.

I also called Dr. Emil Frei, the director and physician in chief at the Dana-Farber Cancer Institute in Boston. Dr. Frei, known to his friends as Tom, was a giant among cancer researchers, widely hailed for his innovations in chemotherapy. Among other achievements, he and his colleagues were pioneers in development of the first truly effective treatment for childhood leukemia. That and his work on other cancers has saved millions of lives worldwide. A decade earlier, we had endowed a chair at Harvard Medical School in Tom's name. When he mentioned that he planned to be in Los Angeles in a few weeks, we arranged to have lunch at my house.

In the meantime, I spoke to another friend, Deepak Chopra, MD, the author and Ayurvedic medicine advocate. He suggested that Lori and I enroll in a weeklong wellness retreat at the Maharishi Ayurveda Health Center in Lancaster, Massachusetts—less than an hour west of Boston.

At that point—still only days since my diagnosis—I also began speaking with Dr. David Heber, MD, PhD, an expert on nutrition at UCLA. I'd seen some articles about the link between high-fat diets and cancer. So one of my first steps was to stop eating just about everything other than uncooked fruits and vegetables. It wasn't easy—I loved hot dogs, lasagna, french fries, gloppy salad dressings, creamy puddings, and the skin on Kentucky Fried Chicken.

Steve Ross had eaten Coney Island hot dogs his entire life. Like most patients, he didn't want to give up his favorite comfort foods even after diagnosis with a life-threatening condition. He didn't stop eating hot dogs until he became so weak he couldn't digest them. Hot dogs and I also had a love affair going back to my college days. Many late evenings at Berkeley, I visited a campus shrine called Top Dog to wolf down several of their frankfurters or bratwurst on tasty grilled rolls. (That diet didn't change when I was back home in LA for the summer. Lori had a job selling hot dogs in the food court of a department store. When I picked her up after work, she scooped up any remaining on the grill and threw them in a bag for me.)

My diet wasn't just hot dogs. I became a star at breakfast-eating contests in our fraternity kitchen, where they gave me the nickname "bottomless pit." The contests were administered by a "chef" who thought lard was one of the essential food groups. No one matched my ability to pack away prodigious amounts of pancakes with syrup, fried eggs, bacon, and sugary cereal.

Breakfast was just the start. The walk to classes included a stop to pick up "lunch"—hot doughnuts freshly pulled from their bath of frying grease and glazed with frosting. My after-classes snack usually included a giant milkshake and a cheeseburger. Most men on that kind of diet would balloon to three hundred pounds, but I've always had a very high metabolism and weight was never a problem. It wasn't until my third semester at Berkeley that I exceeded 150 pounds.

When we moved to Philadelphia after college, I became a devotee of Philly cheesesteaks. At my office in New York, lunch—often eaten standing at my desk with a phone pressed to my ear—was typically a couple of corned beef sandwiches, fried egg rolls, or pizza. After we moved back to Los Angeles in 1978, I resumed going to my favorite high school restaurant, Bob's Big Boy. Just the thought of this LA landmark's double cheeseburger with special sauce and fried onion rings makes my mouth water.

Cancer patients endure many physical insults—loss of hair, drugs that make them look and feel sicker, painful procedures and more. Most doctors, however, don't give them much information about nutrition and many patients can't or won't change their diets. At the time, I had no idea if it would help, but figured it wouldn't hurt me to give up junk food. No hot dog is worth dying for.

*   *   *

A WITCH'S BREW

The MD Anderson conference was an opportunity for more advanced diagnostic tests. By the time Andy von Eschenbach examined me in his clinic, all the news had been bad. The prostate biopsy dashed my initial hope that something other than cancer produced the high PSA reading. The hope that it was a weak tumor was dashed by the "very aggressive" Gleason scores. The hope that surgery offered a cure seemed lost by the finding of lymph node involvement. Step by discouraging step, options were closing. One remaining hope was that the swollen lymph nodes had contained the cancer, preventing metastasis to my bones. If cancer had infiltrated the bone marrow, my prognosis would be even worse.

Andy referred me to an MD Anderson colleague, Christopher Logothetis, a medical oncologist who would oversee a bone marrow test. Fortunately, Chris was able to give me the first good news I'd heard in weeks: "Your bone marrow is clear."

That report gave me a bit of hope. It didn't last long. The next morning, I sat in the audience listening to a prominent cancer researcher explain in technical terms the options for treating metastatic prostate cancer. Projected on the screen behind him was a huge image of a human prostate. At this point, I hadn't fully accepted that my case could be terminal—at least not for many years, perhaps decades. Then the speaker put up a slide describing a subset of patients with high Gleason scores, like mine, whose cancers, like mine, had spread to their lymph nodes but not invaded their bones. It showed the statistics on survival: twelve to twenty-four months with a median of eighteen months.

Eighteen months! I have to get out of here and get some air.

Returning to my room, I needed to lie down, maybe rest for the next twenty-four hours and contemplate what was starting to look like a short, bleak future. But if I had only eighteen months, possibly as few as twelve, I might as well take full advantage of this gathering of experts. After the formal program, I met with an all-star strategy team that included Andy von Eschenbach, Chris Logothetis, Skip Holden, and Snuffy Myers. We talked until late in the evening.

Snuffy, who had special expertise in clinical pharmacology, was well-known for his work devising protocols for investigational cancer drugs. After Andy and Skip described my clinical profile in detail, Chris and Snuffy debated just how hard they could attack my cancer without killing the patient. It was both scary and fascinating. Snuffy's recommendation was to try an experimental drug cocktail that included suramin, an old treatment for parasitic infections like African sleeping sickness. Some medical centers were running early-stage trials to see if it might work against cancer. I asked if it had any serious side effects and Snuffy said no, not really.

At that point, Chris and Andy mentioned there actually were several adverse effects that had been reported in the literature. "Are these effects temporary?" I asked. "Uh . . . not exactly." Snuffy's expression was pained. "It might knock out your adrenal glands, damage your liver and kidneys, and leave you feeling a lot older. Also, some minority of patients risk going into cardiac arrest. On the other hand, it could save your life." Thus, I learned that to many researchers and some clinicians, any side effects that don't kill you are not considered major. Death is major.

I'd have to think very carefully before submitting to a treatment with irreversible effects. Cancer patients undergoing chemotherapy lose their hair, but the hair grows back. This would be permanent.

Early the next morning, I'd been up for a while, going over the options, when a loud knock at the door startled me. Snuffy looked exhausted. "Mike, don't do it!" he shouted. "I've been thinking all night and changed my mind."

It was actually a relief that I wouldn't have to submit to his witch's brew of cytotoxic drugs.* But what else could I do? I pondered that question all day. *Why is this very prevalent disease stuck in the Middle Ages of research? Why isn't the National Cancer Institute driving research toward prostate cancer? What are pharmaceutical companies doing about it? And why are so few scientists focused on it?* I just couldn't understand why there didn't seem to be any organization with the mission of dealing directly with the growing problem of this particular condition.

As the afternoon presentations continued into the evening, it dawned on me that I hadn't heard from anyone who worked at Memorial Sloan Kettering Cancer Center in New York, one of the world's great medical institutions. Just days earlier, I'd spoken to Howard Scher, a renowned prostate cancer specialist at MSKCC. Why weren't he and his colleagues here? "Oh, they're a competitor," an MD Anderson doctor replied. I looked him straight in the eye and said, "Not to patients."

It seemed crazy. These doctors held patients' lives in their hands, yet they had an incomplete picture of the disease without the benefit of expertise from other institutions.†

The more people I spoke to that evening, the more obvious it became that the doctors and scientists at various elite centers viewed one another as competitors, not collaborators. They were all drawing from the same small pool of grant money, and they were all trying to attract revenue-producing patients. It reminded me of when I coached my kids' soccer teams. The biggest challenge was getting the

---

* Although early trials of suramin showed some promise in prostate cancer, it was later withdrawn because of its limited effectiveness and "significant toxicity."

† I thought of this several years later when we expanded our international research program to China. We scheduled a dinner in Beijing to honor award winners from various Chinese medical research centers. But the grant recipients in Shanghai wanted their own separate dinner because they saw the Beijing doctors as competitors.

youngsters to stay in position and cooperate as a team rather than everyone running to where the ball is. Too many medical researchers were running after the same scientific ball and not communicating with each other.

JUST A RAT DOCTOR

One prominent East Coast doctor who attended the conference seemed to be an important physician since all the urologists treated him with great deference. I asked Skip about him and he introduced me: "Mike, I'd like you to meet Dr. Donald Coffey from Johns Hopkins." It turned out that Don Coffey wasn't a physician. As he put it, "I'm just a rat doctor, a PhD. I don't treat people."

Some rat doctor! Widely hailed as "the father of prostate cancer research in America," Coffey held multiple professorships at Hopkins and would later become president of the American Association for Cancer Research. His gentlemanly southern accent and habit of

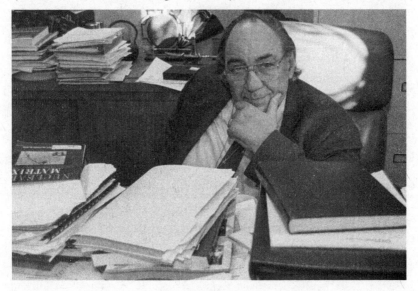

Don Coffey, PhD.

performing magic tricks belied his commanding influence in medicine. He mentored dozens of young scientists and physicians who have gone on to leadership positions nationwide.

I told Don I'd like to come visit him and his medical school colleagues at Hopkins. "Well sure, y'all come on up to Baltimore and I'll show ya 'round." Coffey and other doctors said there were many projects they wanted to undertake, but not enough funding was available from the National Cancer Institute. I'd known NCI director Sam Broder for years—he had helped us establish our early Milken Family Foundation Research Awards—so I made a note to meet with him as soon as possible.

After returning to LA, I immediately made plans for visits to a number of East Coast medical centers and asked Lori to come with me.

First was the Johns Hopkins School of Medicine in Baltimore to reconnect with Coffey and meet some of his protégés. My mission was to learn about the latest medical research advances and to recruit the best young physician-scientists to help us fulfill our goals. Two brilliant early-career doctors I met on that visit were Jonathan Simons and Bill Nelson. Both would go on to produce breakthroughs that changed the course of cancer research history.

When I first met Jonathan, he said his advisors had told him it was "career suicide" to pursue prostate cancer research because there was no money for grants. I told him that grant funding wouldn't be a problem, then added, "You've made the best possible career decision." Jonathan made many original contributions to understanding immunotherapy and the molecular biology of metastasis. Several years later, I recruited him to the Prostate Cancer Foundation, where he served as CEO for fourteen years.

Bill Nelson discovered one of the most common genome alterations in cancer and now heads the Kimmel Comprehensive Cancer Center at Hopkins.

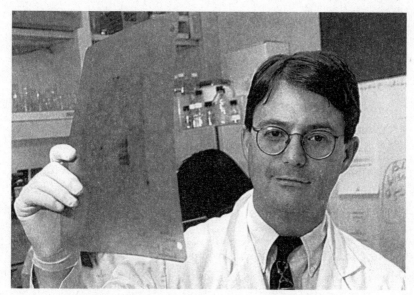

Jonathan Simons, MD, in the early 1990s.

From Baltimore, we made the short drive down I-95 to the Washington Beltway and then the Bethesda exit for the NCI headquarters. Sitting across from Sam Broder, I reviewed more than a decade's work at our Foundation in supporting a wide range of medical research. We'd been giving money, trying to identify the brightest young investigators, and bringing in experts like him to help. But, I told him, it wasn't enough. Perhaps we can get Congress more actively involved. If Sam would agree to speak about the need for more funding, especially for prostate cancer, I would organize a dinner on Capitol Hill. He agreed to speak and to help organize the event.

Then it was up to New York to meet Dr. Howard Scher at Memorial Sloan Kettering Cancer Center. In addition to Chris Logothetis at MD Anderson, Howard was one of the very few medical oncologists whose work was devoted exclusively to prostate cancer.* He and some of his colleagues examined me and scheduled a lymph node biopsy under general anesthesia.

I have a vivid memory of being placed on a gurney for that procedure, rolled down a hall, and spun around like a top before sliding through some swinging doors. There were gurneys everywhere. It brought to mind a day when Lori and I first moved east in 1968. On a trip to New York, we rented a paddleboat for a leisurely ride around the lake in Central Park. It was almost impossible to move because of so many boats. After twenty minutes, we weren't more than six feet from the dock. We might as well have been sitting in a bathtub.

The Sloan Kettering team gave me a sense of optimism. Among other tests, they injected cancer cells from my grossly enlarged lymph nodes into some mice. This was an attempt to create a cell line of my tumor that could act as a target for further therapy. I was rooting for the furry little guys to hang in there long enough to produce actionable data. When the last mouse died, I was crushed.

Despite the failure of the mouse experiment, I had confidence in my medical team's ability to create an effective treatment plan based on the data from all my tests. First was androgen-deprivation therapy, a medical strategy that deprives the cancer cells of the male hormones they need to proliferate. It took several months of this therapy, which involved taking two pills three times a day and getting a monthly injection of Lupron Depot (leuprolide acetate) to bring my PSA count down to the level indicating the cancer was at least temporarily weakened.

Between May and October, the numbers dropped month by

---

* Thanks in part to the Prostate Cancer Foundation (PCF), there are now more than four hundred such specialists. Virtually every major medical center has at least one, and many have several. One of them is Charles ("Chuck") Ryan, MD, who became the PCF's president and CEO in 2021. Chuck sees an important part of his mission to make the PCF the most trusted source of information for tens of thousands of urologists around the world.

month from twenty-four to fifteen, then to ten, five, and three. When they reached zero, I was ready for the next step.

Now another major decision loomed.

THE FANNY MOLD

The choice of whether to add radiation to hormonal therapy is not a decision to be taken lightly. A heavy dose of radiation damages cells and can produce a long list unpleasant effects including nerve injury, urinary and bowel problems, sexual dysfunction, pain, fatigue and, most ominously, future cancers. Some patients choose to do the minimum at the early stages of their treatments. If their PSAs go to zero, they might stop taking hormones in the hope the reading won't go back up; or they might skip radiation. I made the decision to hit my cancer with everything possible: hormones, radiation, diet, lifestyle, even Ayurvedic sesame oil massages, which were invigorating and relaxing.

After researching radiologists to find the best one in Southern California for my case, I chose Christopher Rose, MD. Chris was a leading Los Angeles doctor who was later elected president of the American Society for Radiation Oncology. In 1993, he was among the first to employ three-dimensional, conformal, external-beam radiation. Before this technology was introduced, radiation therapy was two-dimensional; it could only be aimed in the general area of a cancerous mass. That damaged a lot of surrounding healthy tissue. The new 3D process "conformed" to tumors more precisely by zapping the area from several angles at various power levels. It caused less collateral damage.* The physics of conformal radiation are com-

---

* The field of radiation oncology has advanced greatly since 1993. Today's therapy is "four dimensional"—the computer controlling the radiation beam is programmed not only to account for three dimensions of angles, but also for any movement created by the patient's breathing.

plex and I didn't want to be the first patient to undergo it before software bugs were worked out. Fortunately, the clinical trials showed it to be relatively safe.

Patients are advised to remain as still as possible during radiation and it helps to be relaxed. I developed my own relaxation routine when the eight weeks of treatments started. It began with a hot shower. I also pureed most foods to put the least pressure on my digestive system—broccoli soup in place of broccoli, for example. Following each session, I meditated to assist cell repair. None of this was medically prescribed, but I thought it might help.[*]

I had to sit in a custom-molded plastic module that immobilized my midsection so the beam would hit me in exactly the right places. It's rather undignified, but I was thankful for such advanced care. For no clear reason, I've kept my customized "fanny mold" to this day.

The goal of the radiation was to eradicate any residual cancer that wasn't eliminated by the hormonal treatment. If these two therapies failed, there were no more consistently effective options. I fully understood the treatments could cause or contribute to other problems down the road. But what choice did I have? With an initial prognosis measured in months, this was no time to worry about possible consequences decades in the future.

BEATING THE ODDS

I returned to Skip's office monthly for an injection and a blood test to confirm my continuing remission. And I stuck to a disciplined diet,

---

[*] I later described some of this regimen in a 1996 speech to the American Psychosocial Oncology Society.

exercise, and relaxation program. Most importantly, I've enjoyed the fantastic good fortune of thirty years with my family, which now includes ten wonderful grandchildren.

FASTER CURES: SELECTED EVENTS AND MILESTONES

1971 President Nixon declares War on Cancer.
1972 Milken family begins support of medical research and public health.
1977 Increased focus on pediatric neurology and cancer research.
1982 Milken Family Foundation (MFF) launched; increases medical research/public health support.
1983 Development of cancer research awards program.
1985 Program development leading to Milken Educator Awards.
1988 First MFF awards in basic, translational and clinical cancer research.
1989 American Epilepsy Society Research Awards sponsored by MFF.
1991 Milken Institute established.
1993 CaP CURE founded.
1995 National Cancer Summit.
1996 Department of Defense expands medical research programs.
1997 FDA Modernization Act.
1998 First annual Milken Institute Global Conference.
1998 March on Washington.
1998 Five-year doubling of the NIH budget begins.
2003 CaP CURE expands to Prostate Cancer Foundation and *FasterCures*.
2007 Milken Institute publishes "An Unhealthy America."
2007 Melanoma Research Alliance launched.
2009 First Partnering for Cures conference. (Becomes Future of Health in 2018.)
2011 Lake Tahoe Retreat: Accelerating Innovation in the Bioscience Revolution.
2011 National Center for Advancing Translational Sciences (NCATS) established.
2012 Celebration of Science.
2014 CDC/Milken Institute Conference on Public Health.
2014 Milken Institute School of Public Health endowed.
2016 VA/PCF partnership launched.
2016 21st Century Cures Act.
2017 First graduates of Int'l Finance Corp./Milken Institute developing nations program.
2020 Milken Institute/*FasterCures*/PCF responses to Covid-19.
2022 Advanced Research Projects Agency-Health (ARPA-H) established.
2022 California Institute for Immunology & Immunotherapy founded.
2024 Milken Center for Advancing the American Dream opens to public.

Note: A more detailed timeline is at www.fastercuresbook.com.

EIGHT

A New Type of Organization

Starting in the 1970s, we'd initiated several programs to advance medical solutions. Yet even before I'd completed my first round of visits to cancer centers in 1993, it was clear we needed a new organization, a new *type* of organization. It was the beginning of what would evolve into the Prostate Cancer Foundation, the Melanoma Research Alliance, and several centers of the Milken Institute including *FasterCures*.[*]

By early March, we came up with a name for our new organization: CaP CURE. The "Ca" stood for all cancers, the "P" for prostate, and CURE for all diseases. From the beginning, we worked not only

---

[*] The Milken Institute center is branded as *FasterCures* (one italicized word). The title of this book is *Faster Cures* (two words) because it refers more broadly to the process of accelerating medical science.

with other cancer groups, but also with non-cancer organizations. The goal was to increase funding for every form of medical research.

Few biomedical research groups had ever been really active in the sense that they organized themselves around the concept of speeding up science itself. Many were conduits for donations from grateful patients or gifts honoring the memory of a loved one. These groups were often run by people whose hearts were in the right place, but who had little experience managing a risk-taking, proactive organization. Many had budgets weighed down by administrative costs. Whatever was left over would go to established research programs within the silos of individual institutions.

CaP CURE's mission reflected our interactions with hundreds of medical and scientific leaders over the previous twenty years. After much thought, a set of basic principles emerged. They defined an organization that would:

+ Recruit the best and brightest scientists and physicians.

+ Focus on the career paths of these young investigators.

+ Require collaboration in place of competition.

+ Build cross-sector ties.

+ Identify the most promising research not funded by the NIH.

+ Eliminate needless bureaucracy.

+ Relinquish intellectual property rights in exchange for speed and administrative costs.

+ Supplement traditional therapies with proven alternative concepts.

+ Generate public awareness.

+ Educate members of Congress.

+ Assure other disease groups that we were a resource, not a threat.

+ Act with urgency.

For two decades, I'd been on the sidelines, absorbing information, encouraging incremental progress and supporting medical scientists. It was time to run onto the playing field, to become the quarterback of a new team.

CHANGING THE PARADIGM

CaP CURE and its successor organizations would eventually play a major role in keeping millions of cancer survivors alive. That would be in the future, however. In 1993 we knew only that previous efforts hadn't worked very well. CaP CURE would have to break the mold by disrupting and enhancing the process.

Over the years, I'd noted that research institutions often acted like sports teams carefully guarding their playbooks so their "opponents" wouldn't know what they were up to. Many researchers were concerned that if they shared the interim results of their work, they might lose credit for breakthrough ideas before publication in prestigious journals.* Fair enough. If their work is that important, they'll find funding elsewhere. We determined to fund leading-edge research by those who were willing to *share* the results of their work.

---

* By enabling researchers to hear feedback on their work quickly, we started a trend that has significantly changed the medical research process. This accelerated the adoption of the "preprint" publishing model that had been launched by physicists at the Los Alamos National Laboratory in the early 1990s. Today, authors in every scientific field post preprints to obtain comments on their work before submission to peer-reviewed journals. This process greatly accelerated progress on the development of vaccines for COVID-19.

That was a condition of our grants. Within six months, nearly all researchers agreed to it.

The next concern was lack of communication among different sectors of the health industry. Many academic researchers pursuing basic science programs didn't communicate well with for-profit pharmaceutical companies developing clinical applications. Government agencies weren't adequately encouraging the translation of potential cures from the laboratory bench to the patient bedside. Existing disease-specific research groups lacked the resources to change this. Many university researchers felt it could stain the purity of their science if they engaged with profit-making groups. Yet our experience with the Milken Family Foundation's cancer research awards showed there were dedicated scientists in every sector from basic science to translational development to clinical applications. We were determined to improve communication and coordination across sectors.

Too many leading academics were leaving nonprofit medical science to join clinical practices or commercial consulting groups. Saddled with debt from long years of training, they were discouraged by the limited funds available from government research grants. In my opinion, whether in business or any other field, the real problem is almost never a lack of financial capital. The scarce resource is human capital. We vowed to recruit the top young talents in the field and compensate them accordingly so they remained focused on research. They had to believe they were on the right career path, a well-funded path.

NINE FEET OF PAPER

Government agencies must be conservative in spending taxpayers' money. If they take too many risks and fail, whichever political party is out of power in Washington will make it a campaign issue. But always doing what is safe is not the most direct path to real break-throughs. We wanted to encourage risk-taking by identifying the most promising research *not* funded by the NIH.

We also wanted to reduce the onerous requirements that government agencies impose for federal grants. Researchers spent up to a third of their time completing applications, often attaching hundreds of pages of documentation. (In one extreme case, an academic medical center submitted a nine-foot-high stack of paper.) That was just the beginning. Once the application was sent, a researcher could wait a year, sometimes two years, for an answer. By that time, the state of the science might have changed. Too bad—federal rules said the money had to be spent as originally proposed.

Government bureaucracy can sometimes impede rapid progress. One day in 1993, NCI director Sam Broder was showing me around his Bethesda, Maryland, headquarters and introduced me to a young investigator working on a project that looked particularly promising. Unfortunately, funding for that program was about to run out. The cost was $250,000 a year. Soon after that, I sent the NCI a check for $250,000 to continue the project for another year. More than six months later, I received a call from an NCI accountant saying they appreciated it, but weren't sure how to accept my grant. I jokingly said other agencies like the IRS knew how to accept my payments. He was not amused and said, "Please don't do it again." It took them three more months to figure it out. Today, there are separate foundations for the NIH and several other government agencies that know how to accept a contribution from an individual.

Researchers said it was futile to devote months developing grant proposals that would be rejected for lack of funds. This reminded me of my early days in finance when young entrepreneurs kept getting rejected for bank loans because they didn't have an established track record.

We decided to make it simple and encourage the world's leading scientists to fill the pipeline with ideas. Send us an application of any length, but we promise to read only the first five pages. If you have statistical validation of your idea, that's fine; but we'll also consider unproven concepts that sound promising. You don't necessarily have to spend the better part of a year developing proof of your hypothesis. Our belief at CaP CURE was that this would attract the brightest, busiest people to submit ideas. We said we'd review applications quickly and provide an answer in no more than sixty days. If the answer is yes, you'll get the money within thirty days after that.

Looking at five pages instead of thousands, we knew we'd miss a lot of information and perhaps fund some less-deserving projects. That was a trade-off we were willing to make because it would accelerate the science. It was a venture philanthropy model that tries many ideas in the expectation that a few will become major breakthroughs.

Another way CaP CURE kept it simple was to trade intellectual property (IP) for speed and administrative costs. Many organizations add complexity to the research process with contracts that specify retention of patents by the funder. These contracts can take more than a year to negotiate and consume up to half the grant funds, leaving much less for actual research. Our goal was to save lives as fast as possible. "Time equals lives" became our motto. So we decided not to slow the process down by negotiating. In exchange for giving up IP, we required that the institutions pay the overhead costs of their researchers so all our grant money would go directly to research. As a result of the successful research we funded, medical institutions have received billions of dollars in later royalties from approved drugs.*

---

* The cancer landscape has changed since the 1990s when there were fewer cancer studies. In 2014, the Cystic Fibrosis Foundation sold royalty rights for $3.3 billion, a windfall that greatly expanded their capacity to sponsor future research. Now other disease-specific organizations, including the Prostate Cancer Foundation, are rethinking their early financial models.

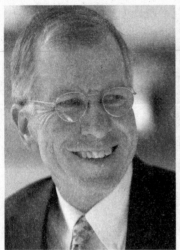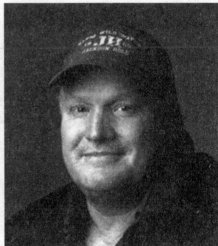

Economists Robert Topel and Kevin Murphy.

We produced hard facts to justify research spending. Helping make the economic argument were Milken Institute senior fellows Kevin Murphy and Robert Topel, protégés of Nobel Prize winner Gary Becker at the University of Chicago.* Their rigorous research showed that increases in longevity since 1970 had added $3.2 *trillion* a year to national wealth, equivalent to half the average annual GDP over that period. Looking to the future, they claimed that a cure for all cancers would be worth $50 trillion.

---

* Professors Topel and Murphy, who have won numerous awards for economic research, jointly wrote the frequently cited 2006 paper "The Value of Health and Longevity," published in the *Journal of Political Economy*. This won the prestigious Arrow Award for the best research paper in health economics in 2007. They showed that the cumulative gains in life expectancy since 1900 were worth more than $1.2 million to the average American in 2000. They also noted that a mere 1 percent reduction in cancer mortality would be worth $500 billion.

A SENSE OF URGENCY

We also launched sophisticated marketing and promotion programs and found celebrity spokespeople for cover stories in magazines. Their stamp of approval was important because for most of the twentieth century, cancer had been something shameful that wasn't discussed in polite company, especially cancers that involved the reproductive organs.

We'd have to change the culture and, as with everything else, we had to do it quickly and creatively. One challenge we faced, particularly in prostate cancer, is that men are less likely than women to ask their doctors for diagnostic tests. Even in men's diseases like prostate cancer, women are often the most active voices for their husbands, fathers, and brothers. I thought back to the mid-1970s when my father was too busy serving his clients to have a doctor check a persistent sore on one of his toes. Finally, my mother insisted he get it checked. Only then did he learn he had melanoma, a condition that eventually metastasized and led to his death.

Advocates for AIDS and breast cancer research had already gained recognition. We noted that they'd been effective with legislators responsible for health agency budgets. Prostate cancer, the most common non-skin cancer in America, was a backwater of medicine by comparison. Yet a man is one-third more likely to get prostate cancer than a woman is to get breast cancer.*

---

* The burden of prostate cancer is not limited to the United States. CaP CURE's research programs, and later those of the Prostate Cancer Foundation, have been international almost from our founding. The first awards outside the United States were made in 1994. Today, grants are made in twenty-eight countries. The PCF Global Research Council, chaired by the internationally renowned oncologist Philip Kantoff, MD, provides objective outside advice.

We wanted other advocacy organizations to understand we weren't trying to grab their piece of the pie. Our strategy was to show this wasn't a zero-sum game—we could increase the size of the pie for everyone. The goal was to double federal funding for research on all life-threatening diseases, triple cancer research, and achieve a tenfold increase in prostate cancer funding.

Our message to other disease foundations was that we needed them to join us in order to increase the funding for everyone. Rather than divert money, we would make the investments required to build new research pathways—new bridges from basic science to translational research to clinical medicine. Once these pathways were shown to work, the results would be available to everyone at no cost. Finally, to assure that happened, we would convene best-practices gatherings to share everything we learned.

In those days before the rise of social media, CaP CURE raised awareness, encouraged diagnostic testing, and sought contributions through both traditional and nontraditional techniques. One example was a partnership with Safeway supermarkets, which had more than 1,500 stores in North America. Under the leadership of Steve Burd, Safeway's CEO, the company worked closely with us to devise what was then a unique fundraising program.

Many nonprofit organizations will tell you it's not worthwhile to solicit contributions of less than ten dollars because it costs them more than that to collect and process each one. Safeway and CaP CURE figured out how to do this for mere pennies. The key was to ask shoppers if they would like to support cancer research with a contribution of one dollar or more at the moment they were about to pay for their groceries. The amount was then added to the grocery checkout total. At several promotional events around the country, I joined other CaP CURE staffers in the role of checkout clerks.

Over several years, the Safeway program brought in some $60 million for CaP CURE's research, much of it through small donations averaging less than two dollars. It was so successful that Safeway expanded our checkout program to raise several hundred million dollars for research on other diseases.

JUST THE BEGINNING

All this activity was quite ambitious. Skip Holden and many others initially had doubts about whether it could work. But they were energized by the opportunity to address life-threatening diseases on a global scale instead of one patient at a time. And they were inspired when we acted with urgency as if lives depended on it. Because they did.

NINE

Getting Up to Speed

———

John Cage, the twentieth-century musical pioneer, once said, "I can't understand why people are frightened of new ideas. I'm frightened of the old ones." In 1993, it seemed to me there weren't nearly enough new ideas in the cancer field. Many existing therapies were either weak or toxic, and few researchers were applying for grants. When applications were received by the NIH or private foundations, there were too few people qualified to review them. As a result, not many grants were being funded, leading to a vicious cycle where few investigators entered cancer research. In fact, at that time, only about 10 percent of the world's leading bioscientists had ever worked on cancer. If we could make more money available, there would be more investigators.

From my previous experience with breast cancer, epilepsy, multiple myeloma, glioblastoma, and other conditions, I knew that government support of research on all diseases was insufficient to drive rapid progress. The statistics on prostate cancer were especially discouraging. At the time, government funding for that disease totaled about $250 per man diagnosed. This compared with more than $1,400 per breast cancer case and tens of thousands for every AIDS case.

Researchers at different medical centers rarely shared their findings. Few of these centers had a well-developed program of prostate cancer research. There was little coordination of the few clinical trials. Human tissue—tumors, skin, and blood—was mostly unavailable to researchers. Not surprisingly, medical school graduates looking for resident fellowships were discouraged from pursuing cancer specialties.

Most public figures who were stricken with prostate cancer kept quiet about it. The disease was "in the closet," as breast cancer had been a generation earlier before women like Betty Ford and Happy Rockefeller spoke out. Many men even hid the diagnosis from their families.*

As part of my research, I explored places in the world where the incidence and mortality of prostate cancer was lower. Countries where a plant-based diet had been predominant—including several Asian nations—had fewer cases. Curiously, there were some US states, mostly in the south, where death certificates almost never indicated prostate cancer as a cause of death. What, I wondered, was the secret to these apparently healthier populations?

Further investigation revealed the true cause of such statistical anomalies—doctors in some areas never listed cancers that involved

---

* That situation changed following publicity about people like Andy Grove, General Norman Schwarzkopf, and me. The late Senator Bob Dole was especially helpful to our cause. Senator Dole didn't let a known diagnosis of prostate cancer impede his run for the presidency in 1996. He spoke out forcefully at our events to raise awareness. In 2003, while running for president, Senator John Kerry was diagnosed with prostate cancer and returned to the campaign trail following surgery. Another presidential aspirant, Mitt Romney, had prostate surgery several years after his candidacy.

the reproductive organs. They held to the Victorian idea that this was something shameful, not to be discussed in polite company, possibly even an indication of sexual deviancy. This was more than foolish—it was dangerous because prostate is among the most inheritable of all cancer types. Men with an affected father or brother are twice as likely to develop prostate cancer as men with healthier relatives. Siblings and children of the deceased would be denied important information about their increased familial risk.

Before CaP CURE, there were no well-known private organizations working on prostate cancer. Many people didn't even know how to pronounce the name of the disease. The word "prostate" was so uncommon that the spell-check feature of Microsoft Word corrected it to "prostrate."

STREAMLINING THE PROCESS

By late spring of 1993, Skip Holden had started our competitive research awards program and organized a review board of leading scientists and physicians to screen the applications. I recruited a diverse group of experts in a range of fields to our board of directors. Seven of our initial twenty-one board members were women.

We received eighty-six grant applications that summer and soon announced the first thirty awards. In choosing which applications should be funded, the review board wanted to encourage novel approaches. They identified a number of promising therapeutic strategies including:

+ Antiangiogenesis (cutting blood supply to tumors);

+ Vaccines and gene therapy;

+ Nutritional studies;

+ Apoptosis (the process of cell death); and

+ Therapies targeting the androgen receptor.

One of our goals was to do preliminary proofs of concept for novel ideas that hadn't been sent to the National Cancer Institute. Our mission was different from the NCI's. Some of the researchers told me later they wouldn't have bothered with that agency's laborious application process, especially since the probability of funding was small. Our streamlined process and openness to new ideas stimulated their creativity. (A few years later, we expanded the list to seventeen priorities with immunology near the top.)

Our sense of urgency strengthened whenever we encountered desperate patients who felt they'd exhausted all treatment options. We approached pharmaceutical and biotechnology industry leaders to encourage greater investment in cancer research. I argued that medical costs were the largest and fastest-growing sector of the economy, that our population is aging, that cancer is a major problem getting worse, and that they should focus on it because only for-profit companies can actually bring products to market.

One day in 1993, I spoke to David Baltimore, the Nobel laureate, who was on the board of directors of Amgen, a major biotechnology company. I told David my concern about so few cancer investments and suggested the company should be spending substantially more—at least $300 million a year—in the area of oncology research. He said I should go see Amgen's chairman, Gordon Binder, whom I'd known for several years. So I drove to the company's nearby headquarters and made the pitch to Gordon. "Mike, you're my friend," he replied. "But I'm running a public company and have an obligation to shareholders." He told me not enough good basic research was coming out of universities and government science centers to justify development of new cancer drugs. Other CEOs echoed Gordon's view.

Over the next two years, we continued to make our case. When I returned to Amgen in 1995, Gordon told me that the basic academic research had increased and they would be dramatically increasing their allocation to cancer drug development. They might have made those investments if I hadn't approached Gordon, but perhaps I was able to start the thought process. The company has since made enormous progress benefiting cancer patients and has now become the world's largest biotechnology enterprise. (In 2022, the FDA approved the Amgen drug Lumakras, which offers new hope for patients with non–small cell lung cancer.)

Many other biotech companies understood the need, but had difficulty raising capital to pursue their ideas. This fact became painfully obvious to me during a presentation at a CaP CURE Scientific Retreat at Lake Tahoe in the late 1990s. I remember sitting in the audience and seeing a shocking slide presented by Mark Simon, then the bioscience division head at Robertson Stephens investment bank. Mark began by citing the small biotechs' insatiable capital requirements. Collectively, 180 companies in the biotech industry were spending more than four times as much on research as Merck, then the largest pharmaceutical firm. Yet the market capitalization of Merck exceeded the combined value that investors had put on the 180 largest biotechnology companies.

The small biotechs had a fantastic future, yet they weren't able to secure enough capital for cancer studies. Most of their programs were in other areas. So we decided to create a road map to show them the potential return on investment in cancer research. I spoke to CaP CURE's directors, most of whom joined me in putting up money for a new venture fund that would invest only in cancer.

Domain Associates, a leading venture capital firm, had deep experience in bioscience investing. The head of Domain, Jim Blair, agreed to oversee and advise the new fund, which we launched in 1998 as ProQuest Investments. We wanted to show that "doing good" could be good business. Once we demonstrated that cancer research investments could produce attractive rates of return, other investors began to move into that space. It helped start a trend toward far greater financial commitments to oncology. Today, hundreds of well-funded biotechnology companies are pushing out the frontiers of cancer research and many of them have been financially successful.

CREATING CENTERS OF EXCELLENCE

We faced many other challenges when we started. On June 17, 1993, the *New York Times* carried an article about prostate cancer with a gloomy conclusion:

> *No evidence exists to show that aggressive efforts to diagnose and treat this [prostate] cancer has had any effect in improving survival.*

Perhaps one reason was the fact that many of the leading US medical centers, although strong in most disease areas, were not really centers of excellence in prostate cancer.* Consider Harvard, for example, home to one of the elite medical complexes in the world. When Harvard executives learned they didn't have a competitive program for the most common cancer in American men, they seemed

---

* Soon after establishing CaP CURE, we urged the NCI to expand SPORE grants for all cancers. SPOREs—Specialized Programs of Research Excellence—support innovative, multidisciplinary translational research approaches that may have an immediate impact on cancer care and prevention. They clearly affirm that a medical center has "made it" to the elite circle of the world's best in an organ-specific research area. The result of our campaign for more SPOREs was dramatic. In 1992, the year before CaP CURE's launch, there were only two prostate cancer SPOREs. A dozen years later, there were eleven such SPOREs, the most of any cancer. The total of SPOREs for all diseases grew from nine to sixty-two over the same period.

unconcerned. I pointed out that they *should* be concerned if only because prostate cancer was going to affect their wealthy donors, who would then turn to other institutions for treatment. I suggested they ask donors to rank their medical concerns. They were shocked when a survey showed prostate cancer was the number two concern on a long list of diseases. (Back pain was the top concern.)

Researchers at Harvard-affiliated hospitals and research institutions had submitted few applications for our first competitive awards in 1993. After the survey of donors, applications picked up, and in 1995 they sent us more applications than any other university center.

Harvard wasn't the only top-tier institution not living up to its potential. The University of California–San Francisco (UCSF) is the only campus in the UC system dedicated exclusively to health sciences. We wanted to help UCSF become a true center of excellence, especially in prostate cancer. To do that, they would need to retain their finest physician-scientists and recruit new leaders in the field. Unfortunately, the opposite appeared about to happen. Memorial Sloan Kettering Cancer Center in New York was searching for a new head of urology and one of their top candidates was Dr. Peter Carroll, an internationally known urologic oncology specialist at UCSF.

We assembled a group with UCSF connections to meet at Lake Tahoe during the 1997 CaP CURE Scientific Retreat. Included were CaP CURE directors Art Kern and Andy Grove, both members of the UCSF governing board. Andy was a prostate cancer survivor and the chairman of Intel. Also participating were the university chancellor, several senior biomedical researchers, and the lieutenant governor of California. I told them that if UCSF lost talent like Peter Carroll, it would be a severe blow. At the time, they were not the leader in prostate cancer, but with Peter, they had a good chance to move up. Without people like him, wealthy patients in Silicon Valley and San Francisco might go elsewhere for treatment and would be less like to make charitable gifts. That threatened to further reduce the quality of their research.

After listening to our presentations, the UCSF directors made a strong commitment to Peter including a broad expansion of their cancer programs. Following that commitment, we helped them with both a restructuring of their research and a fundraising campaign that brought in substantial private funds. Today, UCSF is not only one of the premier cancer centers in the world, but also a leader in prostate cancer.

Meanwhile, Sloan Kettering did not lose out—they successfully recruited Baylor University's Peter Scardino, a great surgeon who helped propel cancer research in New York and nationally. More than a top doctor, Scardino is a strong communicator who looks like he was chosen from central casting. He later joined me on television to deliver important consumer information about cancer.

Closer to home, in 1996, I met with Dr. Gerald Levey, who was then dean of the UCLA School of Medicine and vice chancellor of UCLA medical sciences, which included the hospital and research laboratories. Like those at Harvard and UCSF, the faculty across UCLA's many departments and institutes included a wealth of top-notch scientists. Few of them were focused on prostate cancer.

I asked Gerry if he would convene the university's most talented bioscience researchers. We sought innovative thinkers, even if they had never pursued work in cancer. It was simply a matter of getting the right people together. If we liked their ideas, we'd recruit them.

Several top scientists who were then at UCLA—including Charles Sawyers, Owen Witte, and Arie Belldegrun—participated in these meetings and went on to make transformative contributions in drug development and clinical care. We provided initial funding for their cancer work.* The process has shown me that you can learn a lot by asking a major university to assemble a meeting of their best people in any field even if you don't recruit them.

DOING GOD'S WORK

Successes like UCSF and UCLA started to come after we'd been operating for a few years. Back in 1993, however, the challenges were daunting. The $2 billion federal budget for research on all types of cancer was about half the cost of a single aircraft carrier. Funds for prostate cancer were almost nonexistent. We needed to create awareness, especially on Capitol Hill.

That November, we hosted a "call to action" awareness-raising dinner in the ornate Mansfield Room of the US Capitol. We wanted to showcase the importance of increasing research spending. Another purpose was to celebrate underappreciated scientists by bringing them together with congressional leaders. Support of our competitive research award winners is never just financial—we also recognize their achievements with special events.

Late that afternoon, we assembled our first group of award winners for a photo in front of the Capitol. Andy von Eschenbach recalls the moment:

> I'll never forget walking up the Capitol steps and seeing that beautiful light on the dome and the gleaming white marble. I couldn't believe that this kid from South Philly was walking into the Capitol

---

* We pursued similar interactions with several other medical centers by holding board meetings at Weill Cornell Medicine and Memorial Sloan Kettering Cancer Center in New York, and the Fred Hutchinson Cancer Research Center in Seattle in addition to UCSF and UCLA. In each case, we invited the institution to bring in their most talented scientists to meet with our board members.

of the United States of America and actually going to have dinner there. I only wish that my dad, who died from prostate cancer, could have been there with me. But in a way he was.

Dinner attendees included US senators William Cohen, Bob Dole, Dianne Feinstein, Jake Garn, John Glenn, Richard Shelby, and Ted Stevens. Also the Speaker of the House, Tom Foley; columnist Robert Novak; entertainer and record producer Quincy Jones; NCI Director Sam Broder; the legendary Dr. Emil Frei; and more than fifty other researchers from major medical centers.

I told the audience how irrational it was to spend $100 billion *caring* for cancer patients, but only $2 billion trying to *cure* them. "This is not an intellectual game," Broder added. "It's a matter of life and death."*

The financial markets were already starting to cut drug company stock prices after concluding that Congress might be about to regulate their rates of return like utility companies. Addressing the members of Congress in the room, I said that under that kind of regulation, companies would slash their research budgets and work only on the safest projects. They would no longer be engines of progress. In the four months following that evening's dinner, the value of the ten largest pharmaceutical companies fell by more than $70 billion even as the broader stock market rose. The shares of Merck, which had only recently been named America's most admired company by a business magazine, dropped 25 percent. These companies had become pariahs in a matter of months. Gordon Binder, the Amgen chairman, expressed the industry's frustration: "We thought we were doing God's work!"

Later, when it became clear that the most drastic regulatory proposals would not go into effect, pharma stocks recovered much of

---

* Transcripts of these talks, and many others, are at www.fastercuresbook.com.

their value. But the die had been cast and it forever changed the industry. Innovation suffered as the large companies cut research and focused more on manufacturing, distribution, and marketing. They started merging and buying smaller companies. More research shifted to young biotechnology firms.

"YOU DO THE SCIENCE"

One purpose of the Mansfield Room dinner had been to show our first group of award winners that we appreciated their outstanding work. Continuing that recognition, the next day we took them a hundred miles southwest for a strategy session at the fourteen-thousand-acre Charlottesville, Virginia, farm of John Kluge.* Almost a decade earlier, I'd arranged what was then the largest public financing in the history of securities markets for Metromedia, a company Kluge had founded. As a prostate cancer survivor, John was happy to host an event that could advance the cause of research.

During our discussions in Kluge's home, several of the doctors talked about the frustration and distraction of constantly searching for the next grant to continue their research. I found it frustrating as well—what a terrible misuse of talent. Finally, I stood up and said something to make sure we all understood our priorities moving forward: "Your job is to do the science," I told them. "My job is to raise the money."

This was obviously a new and welcome model for these brilliant doctors who were wasting at least a third of their time searching for funding. The way I saw it, CaP CURE should be able to increase

---

* Kluge (pronounced *KLOO-ghee*) was, at one point, the wealthiest person in the United States. Following prostate cancer surgery, he sought ways to energize his immune system. As I had, he adopted some principles of Ayurvedic medicine including sesame oil massages. He also became close to my neurosurgeon friend Neal Kassell.

their productivity as much as 50 percent by giving them back a third of their time to add to the two-thirds they spent doing research.

In nearly three decades since then, our fundraising for research has made good on that pledge. The money is necessary, but as I said that day in 1993 and have always reminded people since, even more important than the money is the need to recruit the best people and foster a culture of collaboration. That change would start with young investigators.

TEN

Focus on the Young

———

Never have I felt as patriotic as on July 28, 1984. Lori and I stood proudly in the Los Angeles Memorial Coliseum for the opening ceremonies of the Games of the XXIII Olympiad. President Reagan officially opened the games in front of ninety-two thousand cheering attendees and a global television audience of billions. It was incredibly moving—flags waving, music by Gershwin, American athletes leaping with excitement as they circled the field.

A few days later, we saw the American sprinter Carl Lewis fly down the hundred-meter track. He won a gold medal in less than ten seconds. Imagine the lifetime of preparation that goes into those ten seconds of achievement.

Unless they earn a Nobel Prize, medical scientists rarely receive the recognition of Olympic athletes. But they train just as long, often fifteen years starting in college, for the opportunity to work toward lifesaving breakthroughs. That training goes into every new laboratory discovery, every clinical diagnosis.

Since the 1970s, we've advanced the careers of well over six hundred early career researchers. We call them young investigators, or YIs. They work in two dozen countries through the programs of Milken Family Foundation, CaP CURE, the Prostate Cancer Foundation (PCF), *FasterCures*, and the Melanoma Research Alliance (MRA). It's been a great investment.

FUNDING A WINNEBAGO

The very first of these researchers was Steve Rosenberg, who is now a trusted advisor and friend. Steven A. Rosenberg, MD, PhD, joined the National Cancer Institute about the time President Nixon declared War on Cancer. An outstanding physician/scientist, he could have had his pick of lucrative jobs in industry or private practice, but he enjoyed the cutting-edge research atmosphere at the NCI. It was an opportunity to provide hope for patients suffering from the most intractable cancers.

I first met Steve in the early 1980s when we were seated together at a dinner event. As we chatted about research and our families, I asked if he had any summer vacation plans. He said he hoped to rent a recreational vehicle and take his wife, her mother, and his three daughters across the country visiting national parks. Unfortunately, because of his modest government salary, Winnebago rentals exceeded his budget. I told him that joining the NCI shouldn't require a vow of poverty and we would figure out a way for him to make the trip with his family.

Several years before our meeting, Steve was a medical resident at the Peter Bent Brigham Hospital in Boston. One day he encountered a patient whose medical history included surgery for stomach cancer twelve years earlier. The surgeons had closed his abdominal incision saying there was nothing more they could do for him because the cancer had spread so widely throughout his body. More than a decade later, with no treatments, his cancer had disappeared. "Spontaneous regression is one of the rarest events in all of medicine," Steve noted. "But it planted the seed within me that somehow the body had the properties to get rid of a cancer."

That seed of curiosity helped propel extraordinary breakthroughs in cancer immunology. His pioneering work led to the world's first successful gene therapy that harnesses the body's own immune system to shrink tumors. It also put him on the cover of *Newsweek* magazine.* Today, as chief of surgery at the NCI, he hasn't slowed down. But now he looks forward to taking his *grandchildren* on a road trip.

YOUNG INVESTIGATORS

In our early philanthropy, we made many grants to distinguished researchers in recognition of their past breakthrough discoveries. As I've noted, these were effectively lifetime achievement awards. Over time, however, our experience clearly showed that the highest social rate of return on our charitable giving was from investments in early-career physicians and scientists.

The idea that young investigators most often propel science is not

---

* Following the *Newsweek* publicity, Steve was unfairly and inaccurately criticized by some who said he had made exaggerated claims of a cancer cure. He made no such claims. They were made by my friend and client, Dr. Armand Hammer—philanthropist, art collector, diplomat, and chairman of Occidental Petroleum—who supported Steve's work, but overstated the impact of his immunology therapies. We had funded Dr. Hammer and his cancer research organization, Stop Cancer. Steve has mentored many younger researchers in immunology who have gone on to distinguished careers.

new: James Watson, at age twenty-five, was the first to explain the structure of DNA; Albert Einstein was twenty-six when he published the special theory of relativity; Madame Curie developed the theory of radioactivity at age twenty-eight and won the first of her two Nobel Prizes eight years later; Jonas Salk was thirty when his work on polio was funded. As the Nobel laureate Pearl S. Buck once said, "The young do not know enough to be prudent. They attempt the impossible, and achieve it, generation after generation."

Cancer, once a fatal disease in most cases, is now increasingly manageable. In America alone, more than fifteen million cancer survivors live normal lives. Since we established CaP CURE in 1993, the death rate from prostate cancer has fallen 52 percent; and because it had been expected to *increase* with the aging of baby boomers, that rate is actually 80 percent below the NCI's projections. Hundreds of our young investigators produced much of the gain.

Among all of these, some five hundred received support from CaP CURE and the Prostate Cancer Foundation.* By the time they're chosen for the program, each distinguished medical scientist has been in training for nearly half of his or her life. On the way, they earn an MD or PhD degree, or both. Mostly younger than thirty-five, they've achieved postdoctoral or junior faculty positions and focused their goals on a specific area of basic, translational, or clinical research.

It's important to note that these young investigators are working toward breakthroughs that apply to multiple forms of cancer (and often to other life-threatening conditions). PCF support doesn't limit the results of their research to any one disease. Our research grants have helped discover mutations and therapies in dozens of cancer types. The PCF research and clinical communities have also been leaders in the response to COVID-19.

---

* The awards for their investigations go to the medical institutions, which are required to match our support of their laboratory work, provide lab space, and mentors.

Many of our former YIs are now international research and development leaders mentoring a new generation. While it's difficult to put a dollar value on their contributions, the enormous return on past human capital investments seems obvious. It's wonderfully gratifying to meet these gifted physicians and scientists, to hear their stories and learn details of their progress toward cures. They are changing the world through the medical centers they now lead.

We supplement the institutional funding and mentoring each YI receives, not just with financial support, but also with something greater: a community, an opportunity to network, and perhaps most valuable, the chance to mentor the next generation. In the words of Dr. Howard Soule, the PCF's chief science officer, "We create a community they want to belong to because it propels their careers." The best of the best are invited to participate in our annual scientific retreats. Howard notes that "this ticket is not given freely; you have to earn it with participation in cancer research, and the knowledge that you'll support those coming up behind you." If you're invited back, it means your career is on track.

Young Investigator Awards help advance the careers of these doctors and scientists. We select them through a competitive peer review process by a jury of top cancer researchers. Typically, an award would be for $300,000 over three years, although some investigators have banded together to apply for multimillion-dollar team-science awards.

The scientific and social return on this investment has been astounding. Once our awardees prove a concept, follow-on grants from government and industry typically leverage the original investment nearly tenfold. The American Society of Clinical Oncology (ASCO) regularly invites dozens of PCF early career researchers to make presentations at its annual conference, one of the most important events in cancer research.

Most importantly, thanks in substantial measure to their work, the FDA has approved twenty-three drugs for prostate cancer compared to only three when we launched CaP CURE in 1993. In fact, attendees at our scientific retreats over the past three decades have been involved in development of almost every prostate cancer treatment advance.

CREATING A COMMUNITY

The underlying principle of supporting young investigators is the same as in our programs for Milken Scholars, teachers who win a Milken Educator Award, or participants in the International Finance Corporation-Milken Institute Capital Markets Program: provide a community that will advance their careers. It's essential for the YIs to know they're not alone, that there are others out there, facing the same challenges, wrestling with a particular problem. Not every day can be a good day; not every experiment will work out; progress might be stymied for a time. But the family of colleagues is always there. Data gets you only so far. You need to understand these investigators at a deeper level. You need to know their stories.

I wanted to know the story of a scientist I met several years ago during a tour of a cancer research laboratory. He told me he was considering an offer from a company that hoped to produce better fruit. They wanted him to conduct research on the genomes of apples. I said it might be better if he stayed in cancer research even if it meant the world would have to get along with the same apples for the next twenty years. During those two decades, millions of patients could benefit from his work. Fortunately, he didn't leave his lab and went on to contribute to improved therapies. One of our big challenges today is to convince a generation of students to choose bioscience careers. Apples can wait; patients cannot.

ELEVEN

Speeding the Search

"Let's go for a walk, Chris." I wanted to get Dr. Christopher Logo-thetis away from the other conference attendees so we could review my options for continuing treatment. We'd been meeting all day at the 1994 CaP CURE Scientific Retreat in Santa Barbara's Four Seasons Biltmore Resort.

A red-brick path led from the main hotel building past colorful bougainvillea hedges and perfectly manicured lawns to a walkway along Butterfly Beach. The sun had almost sunk into the Pacific Ocean as seagulls floated overhead. A few of the younger doctor-scientists carried rented surfboards ahead of us.

This interlude between the scientific presentations and dinner was my first chance to spend some time in person with Chris since we'd first met at MD Anderson Cancer Center in Houston a year earlier. My focus wasn't on the idyllic Southern California setting—I was more concerned with figuring out the best ways to stay alive.

In the year since Chris had joined my treatment team, I'd followed an initial hormone regimen and had eight weeks of radiation therapy. Meanwhile, I completed my training with the Ayurvedic doctor who had lived in our house for several months. And I stuck to a disciplined diet of raw fruits and vegetables.

When Chris and I first met, he described his strategy for treating difficult cancer cases as "Keeping you alive long enough until the next therapy becomes available." Now, with the completion of radiation, I asked him what that next therapy might be. "Let's wait and see how you progress after the radiation. Hopefully, the cancer won't return."

I respected Chris, but couldn't accept his answer.

In my opinion, we needed to be more proactive and suggested we figure out what new research programs could be accelerated if they had a higher level of funding. After all, time equals lives and these programs could be worthwhile for future patients even if they didn't produce useful therapies in my lifetime. I was also about to begin a series of international trips to see if there were promising alternatives that could supplement my standard treatments.

ATTACHING A STRING

That 1994 retreat in Santa Barbara was a game changer because of its impact on the cancer community. Compared to our later events, the attendance was relatively small. There were about a hundred registrants, most of whom were university-based American physicians and scientists focused on oncology. About fifteen of the attendees represented biotech companies.

At first, everyone sat with their own little group—academics on one side and the biotechs across the room. Dr. William Fair, the head of urological oncology at Memorial Sloan Kettering Cancer Center, told me he had never gone to a meeting that included corporate people. His practice of not mixing with "the other side" was all too common.

I'd considered creating an assigned seating chart to mix commercial researchers among the academics. Rather than force this integration, however, I decided to let everyone discover their common interests. By the second day, after presentations from some of the industry leaders, people began to mingle. Mutual respect was growing and people were realizing how they could help each other. Academics now saw the value of interaction with for-profit scientists. One speaker told me it was the most exciting event he'd attended in years. Normally, he said, "I see the same old guys trotting out the same old ideas. You bring in folks from different fields. It's like being at the Los Alamos planning meetings working on the Manhattan Project."

My own research combined with the experience of eating a plant-based diet convinced me that sessions on nutrition should be part of the retreat agenda. But others felt if we put too much emphasis on nutrition, some of the leading scientists who didn't consider it "hard science" might be put off and decide not to attend. We had to show that we were very serious about science.

Nearly three decades later, these annual gatherings are a major event on the global scientific calendar. Coveted attendance slots are limited to about 650 of the world's leading medical investigators from a long list of disciplines. Among them are physician-scientists, computational and structural biologists, epidemiologists, radiologists, physicists, biochemists, mathematicians, computer scientists, nutritionists, medical ethicists, and more. They come from more than twenty countries and represent not just academic medical centers, but also pharmaceutical and biotechnology companies as well as disease-specific research organizations and government health agencies.

We hold our annual scientific retreats in quiet settings far from the urban centers of academic and clinical medicine. After hosting the event in Santa Barbara in 1994 and 1995, we moved to the

Nevada side of Lake Tahoe in 1996. With no direct flights and an hour drive over the Sierra Nevada crest, it's not easy to reach. This is intentional—we want attendees to interact with each other and stay focused on the presentations. We stimulate collaboration with people they otherwise would never have met. Each presenter must be prepared to answer tough questions from many of the world's most knowledgeable people in his or her field.*

PASSING THE BATON

Medical researchers are like runners in a relay race. Each carries a baton representing a single line of inquiry, a possible cure. Each hands the baton to another runner as it works its way around the track from basic research to product development to clinical trials and, eventually, to patients.

The problem within medicine is that the runners were each waiting for his or her turn to run, passing the baton from one to the next. If you've ever run track, you know that in an actual race you must begin running your leg of the race well before the runner with the baton reaches you. You want to take the baton while running so the baton passes seamlessly into your hand, and you don't miss a step.

My goal was to make the process of medical breakthroughs more like a race of well-practiced relay racers, moving one possible cure—that baton—quickly from one runner to the next. That's what we started to do in CaP CURE's early days between 1993 and 1998. We established seventeen strategies and started runners going on each of

---

* Because of COVID-19, the 2020 and 2021 Scientific Retreats were held online. Although this obviously precluded in-person encounters, we were able to open the registration to several thousand more professionals from dozens of countries. It remains the foremost scientific conference in the world devoted to prostate cancer.

them at the same time.* In some cases, we began collecting data even before it was clear how the data could be used most effectively.

All these strategies came together and were remixed at our annual scientific retreats. New therapies began to emerge, successful therapies that saved lives. Because we act as a venture philanthropy, our goal is to show proofs of concept so that industry and government will pick up the funding of our original research and leverage it many times over.

Three decades later, the strategies of collaboration and venture philanthropy have clearly had an impact. Of course, in 1993, we didn't know what successes lay ahead. All we had was hope, determination, and a plan. To implement the plan in both the laboratory and the clinic—and the translational process linking them—we needed great physicians and scientists, people like Jim Allison.

PUSHING OUT THE FRONTIERS

Jim grew up in the small town of Alice, Texas, less than two hours by car from the Mexican border. The 1957 Sputnik launch fueled his interest in science. Thanks to Sputnik, the University of Texas offered summer programs in science for high school students.

Jim started college as a premed major at age sixteen. Between listening to the music of Willie Nelson and sneaking down to Mexico with his buddies to hang out in bars, he sometimes went to classes. At first, he thought he might follow in the footsteps of his father, a country doctor who treated patients in the Hispanic part of town

---

* As of 2020, we were monitoring twenty potential research areas, twelve of which have drugs in development. According to estimates by McKinsey & Company, each of these drugs in the pipeline, if approved by the FDA, could save at least nine thousand lives a year in the United States alone.

where they lived. Eventually, he gravitated toward science. Jim once told me why he didn't go into medicine: "MDs fill their heads with facts they've memorized and then draw on those facts in treating patients. They're always supposed to be right. What I love about science is that it isn't about memorizing and trying to be right; in science, you're supposed to be *wrong*, which makes it a lot more fun."

When he was still in college, a biology professor mentioned a new discovery called T cells, which attack foreign substances in the body. Not much was known about these cells and Jim liked the challenge of figuring them out. After years of hard work, he became the first to explain their structure. Several more years in his lab produced checkpoint therapies, one of the most exciting breakthroughs in cancer treatments of the past quarter century. It earned him the 2018 Nobel Prize.

At our 1997 retreat, long before he was well known, Jim said something that changed my entire perspective and mobilized me to focus on immunology. In fact, it was an idea that changed the world. "Your immune system," said Jim, "is smarter than any of us. Disease occurs when it fails." He explained to me there are three reasons people develop cancers:

1. <u>The patient's immune system is weakened by age, lifestyle choices, and past diseases.</u> In the majority of cancers, this causes inflammation, which has become a central focus of cancer research.

2. <u>The cancer sometimes disguises itself so it can compromise the body's defenses.</u> Building on Allison's insight, Dr. Carl June at the University of Pennsylvania later conceived the concept of cellular therapies where a patient's own immune cells, rather than a donor's, are engineered to destroy cancer. The idea is to energize the immune system by removing T cells from the patient, "teaching" those cells how to recognize the disguised cancer cells, and then returning them to the body in "attack

mode." Deploying these chimeric antigen receptors (CAR-T cells), Dr. June successfully improved treatments for acute lymphoblastic leukemia, the most common cancer in children. Then, in 2022, the FDA approved a Johnson & Johnson CAR-T cell treatment for multiple myeloma, another blood cancer. In J&J studies, 83 percent of patients had a complete remission with no detectable cancer cells.* We have funded Dr. June's work for many years.

3. <u>The cancer turns off the immune system.</u> Allison's greatest triumph may be the development of checkpoint inhibitors that turn the immune system back on by suppressing what had turned it off. In other words, Jim figured out how to block the "off" switch.

Listening to Jim, I decided to fund ongoing research at his Berkeley lab. Helped by our initial grant and other funding, Jim was able to demonstrate the market potential of his "immune system off-switch blocker." After further development, Berkeley received initial payments of more than $87 million from Bristol Myers Squibb for Allison's antibody. These funds were plowed back into further research.

In 2011, the Food and Drug Administration approved Yervoy, which had been developed from Allison's work, after clinical trials showing dramatically extended survival times for many patients with advanced melanoma.† And because today's precision medicine

---

* *Wall Street Journal*, February 28, 2022. "FDA Approves Cell-Based Multiple Myeloma Therapy Discovered in China" by Peter Loftus. The treatment is expensive—more than $400,000—but needs to be taken only once and is expected to be covered by insurance. Considering the value of a human life and the alternative cost of lifetime treatments, the price seems more justifiable.

† Checkpoint inhibitors are most effective in cancers where cells mutate rapidly. Melanoma cells multiply quickly and undergo frequent mutations of different types. The growth of prostate cancer is generally a slower process and creates fewer mutations. That's why Allison's initial breakthroughs failed in prostate cancer trials, but were spectacularly successful in melanoma and other fast-growing malignancies.

can identify the specific subtype of a tumor anywhere in the body, Yervoy and similar immunology drugs, such as Keytruda and Opdivo, are now being used against several other types of cancer. Millions of people around the world have benefited from the spin-offs of Jim Allison's breakthrough discoveries.*

NEW THERAPY CHOICES

Another example of the PCF's venture philanthropy model is a drug called Zytiga (abiraterone acetate). Abiraterone is highly effective for men with a common type of prostate cancer that no longer responds to such frontline therapies as hormones, radiation, and surgery. We supported development teams led by Dr. Johann de Bono at London's Royal Marsden Institute for Cancer Research; another group at Seattle's Fred Hutchinson Cancer Research Center; and Cougar Biotechnology, a company founded by Los Angeles–based physician-entrepreneur Arie Belldegrun. In 2009, Johnson & Johnson purchased Cougar, including the rights to abiraterone, for $1 billion. They and others then invested another $1 billion in further development of the drug, which was approved by the FDA in 2011. The PCF had invested $14 million in proving its earlier effectiveness. Just as importantly, we focused other investors on what we considered an important cancer priority. They leveraged our original investment dozens of times over. Today, as one of the most successful cancer therapies, abiraterone is extending millions of lives worldwide.

---

* The promise of immunology continues to create excitement throughout the medical and scientific communities. In late 2022, five major philanthropists and the state of California joined me as founding donors in announcing the California Institute for Immunology and Immunotherapy (CIII), which will be housed on the UCLA campus. We plan this center to be a "field of dreams" that attracts hundreds of scientists from around the world to advance understanding of the human immune system and develop innovative treatments.

CaP CURE and the PCF also provided $13 million in funding for development of Xtandi (enzalutamide), another very important prostate cancer treatment that provides an additional choice for delaying metastatic disease. Xtandi was discovered at UCLA by Charles Sawyers, MD, and Michael Jung, PhD, and then further developed and marketed by Medivation, a specialty drugmaker later acquired by Pfizer for $14 billion.* Dr. Sawyers was one of the scientists we had brought in to present to the CaP CURE board in 1996. That turned out to be a crucial meeting because it focused him on our priorities in cancer.

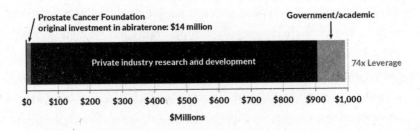

Years later, UCLA chancellor Gene Block called me to ask if we'd be interested in buying the royalties for enzalutamide for more than a billion dollars. I told him we appreciated the opportunity, but we'd pass on it since we had supported the initial research leading to the drug's discovery and, as had been our standard practice, did not retain intellectual property rights. I said we'd reach out to Pablo Legorreta, the chairman of Royalty Pharma, to see if he was interested. He was. Royalty then paid UCLA and the researchers between $1.1 and $1.2 billion for their royalties. The FDA approved Xtandi in 2018 after it was shown that it reduced the risk of metastasis or death by a highly significant 71 percent.

Such successes still underestimate the impact of these research ac-

---

* Dr. Sawyers is now at Memorial Sloan Kettering Cancer Center in New York.

tivities. In fact, the therapies emerging from the CAPCURE/PCF's funding have applicability in *an estimated seventy-three types of cancer.* That's because cancer is no longer thought of as a disease of particular organs—the lungs, breast, prostate, colon, etcetera. We now know there's more complexity to cancer growth than can be found or studied in a single organ site.

There are two aspects to this complexity: First, a single type of cancer, such as breast cancer, may be found in different parts of the body. It's still breast cancer no matter where it emerges. Second, a particular type of mutation is often shared across different types of cancer. Thus, for example, more than 90 percent of colon cancers have a mutation that is often found in prostate cancer.

Furthermore, as former NIH director Francis Collins has pointed out, the genomic understanding being developed today in cancer research will form the basis of progress against *all* human disease. It will, says Dr. Collins, teach us how to treat Alzheimer's and Parkinson's—diseases that threaten to become an enormous social and economic burden.

There are many others like Jim Allison, Arie Belldegrun, Carl June, Charles Sawyers, and Owen Witte among the investigators working on the research projects we've funded. Allison's story highlights the important influence of Sputnik. He and I are close to the same age and we agree that many scientists of our generation chose to go into science at least in part because of Sputnik. That's why we've launched several programs designed to rededicate the nation to bioscience.

PART III

The March of Progress

TWELVE

Expanding the Mission

_____

My previous involvement in medical research combined with the experience of being a patient since 1993 provided a basic understanding of how cures are developed. But I needed to delve more deeply into the research process to become a more effective contributor. My thinking had evolved from someone who was dying of cancer to living with the disease. Not just surviving, but pursuing an energetic role that could have an impact.

Many patients whose initial treatments have driven their PSAs down to zero just want to move on. Hoping for the best, they come back to their doctors only once a year for blood tests and possibly a hormone injection. Some do fine while others receive an unpleasant surprise in their annual test results. Even though my PSA had reached zero by late 1993, I decided to build a monthly checkup and hormone injection into my routine. Once a month for more than twenty years, I'd pop into Skip Holden's clinic on the way to my office. If the month-to-month results showed a significant variation, I'd know about it quickly.

By 1995, our organization had become a recognized force in the medical community. Its innovative strategy of fostering collaboration among the best and brightest researchers was encouraging new disease-specific research organizations to follow our model. Eventually, many long-established groups adopted the same methods.

Many of us still felt that too many patients were dying from cancer without being given an opportunity to try experimental drugs that seemed effective in early testing. During the summer of 1995, I met at Lake Tahoe with General Colin Powell, the former chairman of the Joint Chiefs of Staff (and future secretary of state) and urged him to assume leadership of the cancer advocacy movement. As we discussed how the War on Cancer should proceed, Powell cited the philosophy of the commander on the ground in the 1991 Gulf War, General Norman Schwarzkopf: You never have all the information you need about an enemy, but you have to move forward with the best information and tools available. There was a clear parallel in the use of experimental drugs to treat cancer— if we know a drug provides benefits, we shouldn't wait until we have perfect information before allowing its use for desperately ill patients.

We addressed this issue later that summer by sponsoring a Working Meeting on Standards in Washington to encourage the faster release of cancer drugs. Some fifty representatives from academic institutions, the FDA, the NCI and advocacy communities attended. This effort was to determine if we could treat cancer drugs differently than we treat medicines for back pain, arthritis, and other types of diseases that might have to go to Phase 3 clinical trials to be sure they worked effectively. With some diseases, you can safely withhold treatment for a year. Not so with cancer. Shouldn't patients with short life expectancies be allowed to try a drug that has worked in Phase 2? Our message to the FDA: Let's work as a team to accelerate cancer research.

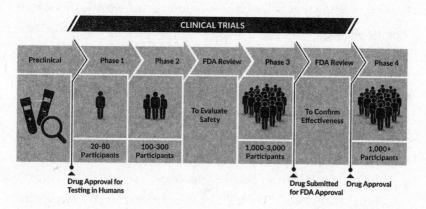

Emil Frei, who had held the Milken Family Foundation chair at the Dana-Farber Cancer Institute, was now the Institute's physician in chief emeritus. He played a leadership role in the standards meeting. A few days later, he wrote:

> *I believe we have formed the basis of a major change in clinical trials and a major improvement and acceleration of progress in cancer treatment. The positive and enthusiastic thrust of CaP CURE is quite in contrast to the pessimistic mood that pervades much cancer research.*

There was encouraging agreement that the process of drug approvals could be improved. The meeting's recommendations were summarized in a white paper that CaP CURE circulated to key decision makers in the administration and on Capitol Hill. But it would take more to turn agreement into action.

PLAN OF ATTACK

We immediately joined with several cancer organizations to plan a broader meeting that fall, a Cancer Summit, that would raise Washington's awareness of how the disease impacted families. The first step in achieving that awareness was to define the problem succinctly. Our central message: Cancer will strike one of every two men and one in three women—more than 100 million Americans. As the date for the summit approached, I jotted down ideas for a keynote speech that would outline specific solutions to that problem. Then I asked Lee Hood to brainstorm with me about these ideas and consolidate them to a shorter list of key points.

Leroy (Lee) Hood, MD, PhD, had been trailblazing the systems biology revolution for decades. In 1986, he devised the automated DNA sequencer that transformed the field of human molecular genetics and genomics; he won the Lasker Award for studies of immune diversity; and now he stood astride the fields of biology, technology, and computation. Impatient with the pace and restrictions of universities, he later founded the Institute for Systems Biology to focus on the most pressing issues in human health through scientific collaborations that stretch across disciplines. We had provided substantial support for Lee's work on the genetics of cancer. At the previous year's CaP CURE Scientific Retreat, he presented a framework for a new genetics consortium.

Lee and I worked late into the night before the Cancer Summit (which was formally called the First National Congress on Cancer Survivorship). We agreed my speech should call for a "rethinking" of the War on Cancer that would move it from a "war of attrition" to a "plan of attack."* After discussing several dozen ideas, we settled on ten of the most important principles:

---

* The full speech text is at www.fastercuresbook.com.

1. Internationalize the War on Cancer;

2. Invest more;

3. Recruit a world-class scientific team;

4. Coordinate worldwide cancer resources;

5. Accelerate technology transfers;

6. Push the technological envelope;

7. Create a world library of organic chemicals;

8. Accelerate approval of new drugs;

9. Get products to market faster;

10. Mobilize patients and families.

Before delivering this speech the next morning, I was scheduled to appear on NBC's *Today Show*. The day's news was dominated by the shutdown of the US government because Congress had failed to pass an omnibus appropriations bill. The press had a field day with that, showing empty office buildings and providing a forum for partisan bickering. Democrats blamed Republicans for holding up the people's business, and Republicans attacked Democrats for budget deficits. As I waited to be interviewed in a hotel hallway outside the summit, the previous *Today Show* guest, Speaker of the House Newt Gingrich, was assailing political opponents for "leaving future generations with the burden of a huge government debt." Moments later, I was on the air telling a national audience we should indeed be concerned about what we leave to future generations. But I wasn't talking about budget deficits.

My parents' generation fought World War II to leave us a better world, free from tyranny, so we could enjoy the benefits of democracy. It is our generation's responsibility not to leave the burden of cancer and other serious diseases to our children.

Soon after that appearance, I was on the stage of the National Cancer Summit to deliver my ten-point speech. Wrapping up the talk, I made an emotional appeal:

We have strived to leave our children a world devoid of war, yet more American lives will be lost in one year to cancer than were lost in all the wars of the twentieth century.

We have strived to leave our children with a country free from debt, yet we are burdening them with massive medical costs associated with an aging population and ever-increasing rates of cancer.

We have strived to leave our children with a world that celebrates and cherishes the sanctity of a single human life, yet we are unwilling to make the financial and moral commitments necessary to lift the burden of cancer from the next generation.

Through sins of omission and commission, we have created a world where one in five will have their lives cut short by cancer. This is too great a burden to leave to our children and grandchildren.

For those children and the children of future generations, let us find a cure for cancer. Let us do it now.

Let us choose life.

Among those who listened to the speech was the new director of the National Cancer Institute, Richard Klausner, MD, who was joined at the summit by every living former NCI director. Klausner had already reviewed the white paper from the previous summer's Working Meeting on Standards and now he had evidence of growing support for action. Soon he was on the phone to President Clinton's healthcare advisors in the White House.

Early in 1996, the president signed an executive proclamation that revised the FDA's review process for experimental cancer drugs to make them more quickly available to patients. "The waiting is over," said Clinton. "We cannot guarantee miracles, but at least hope is on the way." The next year, Congress passed the FDA Modernization Act, which sought to reduce the average time required for drug review. The act streamlined the drug-approval process and expanded access to clinical trials.

NEW PROGRAMS

Our early funding of medical investigators has shown real progress. For example, in 1994, Neil Bander, MD, at what is now Weill Cornell Medicine in New York, produced monoclonal antibodies to PSMA (prostate-specific membrane antigen) that bind to living cells. More than 3,700 research papers following up on Dr. Bander's PSMA discoveries testify to the significance of his original CaP CURE–funded work. The FDA recently approved two new prostate cancer scans developed with CaP CURE/PCF funding that are based on the Bander discovery. The scans provide a far more precise view of suspect cells than is possible with hit-or-miss needle biopsies. On one of my podcasts, PCF-funded investigator Michael Hofman at the Peter MacCallum Cancer Centre in Australia described an important *therapeutic* use of the PSMA protein as a target for precision-targeted radiation. Over the years, we've invested nearly $30 million worldwide in PSMA studies.

As our researchers were pursuing these investigations, I sometimes found myself at odds with highly esteemed medical leaders. In the mid-1990s, Martin Abeloff, MD, was chief oncologist and director of the cancer center at Johns Hopkins. I respected Marty as an elite doctor and administrator who was well liked by his colleagues. But we disagreed on one key point: I said it was possible to accelerate science; he said that was wrong because the scientific process moves forward in careful, incremental steps, one minor breakthrough building on top of another. I cited historical examples—a cholera outbreak, a civil war—that scrambled the old ways of thinking and produced sudden waves of innovation. Sadly, Dr. Abeloff died from leukemia in 2007. If he were with us today, he would see the phenomenal speed with which scientists developed effective vaccines and antiviral therapies for COVID-19. It was a once-in-a-century threat that accelerated science.

In the late 1990s, I participated in a Johns Hopkins School of Medicine graduation ceremony. On the stage with me was William Brody, a radiologist who had been the university's president for several years. He was telling me and all the bright medical students the same things Marty Abeloff had said about the slow, steady pace of progress. These prominent doctors and doctors-to-be knew more than I about the *practice* of medicine; but I had to counter their defeatist view of the medical research *process*. Drawing on my two decades of experience, I spoke passionately about how waiting for incremental fixes can be a death sentence. CaP CURE and other groups like it were determined to speed up the process.

Just look at the leaps forward in medicine that emerged from the American Revolutionary and Civil Wars, World War I, World War II, Korea, and Vietnam. Hundreds of examples include rapid improvements in vaccinations, anesthesia, transfusions, chemotherapy, and frozen blood storage. One interesting advance is the case of intraocular lenses (IOLs). When a patient's natural lens is removed from an eye during cataract surgery, it's now routine to replace it with a tiny artificial plastic lens that restores excellent vision. Before such lenses were perfected in the 1970s, postsurgical cataract patients usually had to wear thick "Coke bottle" glasses.

Early attempts to create artificial lenses failed because the body mounts an inflammatory response to reject foreign objects in the eye. Then Dr. Harold Ridley, a British ophthalmologist, had an inspiration. In World War II, Royal Air Force pilots sometimes suffered eye injuries when the plastic canopies of their planes shattered after being hit by enemy shells. While removing plastic fragments from pilots' eyes, Dr. Ridley realized that the particular type of plastic used in the canopies—poly(methyl methacrylate) or PMMA—was inert. The immune system did not produce an inflammatory reaction. With this discovery, Ridley developed the first implantable lens in the late 1940s. IOL design evolved and by the 1970s, implantation became a standard procedure. (Having had cataract surgery on both my eyes, I can personally attest to its value. I'm one of millions of patients who enjoy clearer, brighter vision with more vivid colors.)

We can't wait for another war to produce accelerated medical advances when patients are dying right now.

DEFENSE

Meanwhile, we were forging ahead with several other initiatives. The first of these involved the Department of Defense. People are sometimes surprised to hear that the DoD has a large cancer research program. Military recruitment advertising shows healthy young men and women in uniform. But as military men and women age, a significant number of them are diagnosed with prostate or breast cancer and many of them die. It occurred to me that the DoD could emulate the biomedical programs of the National Aeronautics and Space Administration, which studied the effects of space flight on the human body. In 1995, I met with NASA Administrator Dan Goldin, who outlined NASA's medical research. I wondered if similar programs could be started in the Defense Department to work on prostate cancer. Perhaps this could be part of the "peace dividend" since America was not involved in any active wars at the time.

Over the next two years, my colleagues and I met with more than one hundred members of Congress to encourage support for increased cancer research. Some of this work was coordinated with advocates for breast cancer research, who were also leading an effort for increased funding by the DoD. CaP CURE board member and Intel chairman Andy Grove also became an effective advocate for the Department of Defense research program.

Between the 1990s and 2022, Congress appropriated more than $4 billion for the breast cancer research program. In late 1996, Congress approved a Defense Department program of prostate cancer research—an initial $45 million appropriation for 1997. Grove and CaP CURE executives then met with Dr. Klausner, the NCI director, to discuss how the NCI's programs could most effectively coordinate with those at the DoD's Prostate Cancer Research Program (PCRP). Since 1997, the PCRP has provided more than $2 billion for peer-reviewed prostate cancer research studies.

SIGN 'EM UP

For many years, researchers had tried to recruit families with a high incidence of prostate cancer to participate in genetic research studies. But it hadn't been easy to find them. In ten years of trying, Johns Hopkins had been able to recruit only ninety such families. I had an idea when I heard about this. I suggested, tongue in cheek, that the Hopkins recruiters use the revolutionary new technology of television. (Actually, TV had been in people's homes for forty-five years.) If we went on TV, we could compress the recruitment time. Back in the early 1980s, I had arranged the financing that allowed media entrepreneur Ted Turner to expand CNN, the Cable News Network. Now maybe CNN could return the favor.

I called Larry King, a longtime friend whose *Larry King Live* reached a nationwide audience every night, and explained that his CNN show could encourage families to sign up for genetic studies. King was not enthusiastic. "Mike, I'd like to help, but it's sweeps week and I can't afford low ratings. We've never done a show on anything as negative as cancer—it's just not an exciting broadcast concept. But go talk to Ted. If he says okay, I'll do it."

Turner approved the show after I promised to assemble a strong panel of guests. On the first in a series of broadcasts, King interviewed General Norman Schwarzkopf (who had recently been diagnosed with prostate cancer), Skip Holden, Lee Hood, and me. Hood explained his new initiative called PROGRESS (Prostate Cancer Genetic Risk Evaluation and Screening Study) that we funded at the University of Washington and the Fred Hutchinson Cancer Research Center in Seattle. It turned out to be one of Larry King's more successful shows. Following the broadcast, more than three thousand people from eighteen countries called the program to learn more about the study. Many who called didn't have prostate cancer but just wanted to help; some even said they saw General Schwarzkopf and were "reporting for duty." As a result, we signed up nearly three hundred families who had three or more close relatives with prostate cancer. Today, of course, it's much easier to recruit people using the internet. Organizations with the reach of Apple, Google, or Facebook can sometimes get tens of thousands of people to sign up for a health program within a day.

GOING TO WAR

All this activity was quickly raising prostate cancer awareness. Hardly a day passed that some publication wasn't calling requesting an interview about what had previously been a little-known threat to men. Many of the reporters had scant knowledge of cancer, however, and the media gave it only sporadic coverage. I decided to meet with Walter Isaacson, then the managing editor of *Time* magazine.

"You have war correspondents covering every conflict around the world," I told him. "But you don't have a correspondent covering the biggest war, the War on Cancer." Walter wasn't all that impressed. He told me their studies indicated that 27 percent of Americans think they've been visited by an alien. "Perhaps," he joked, "we should have a UFO correspondent." Still, I persisted and Isaacson agreed to consider increased coverage.

Some months later, *Time*'s Leon Jaroff called me. "We'd like to do a story about prostate cancer and put you on the cover." It was great that a major magazine finally realized the importance of prostate cancer, and I was happy to tell my story. But I suggested that a cover photo of a war hero like General Schwarzkopf would draw more readers. Within weeks of the Schwarzkopf cover story in the spring of 1996, Andy Grove told the story of his prostate cancer treatment in *Time*'s sister publication, *Fortune*. Grove was candid about the agonizing decisions prostate cancer patients face, the potential for sexual side effects, and the need for patients to assert themselves in interviewing different medical specialists.

Now that it was more acceptable to discuss prostate cancer, awareness of the disease was growing dramatically. The publicity helped increase public knowledge and built a constituency for increased federal research funding of all serious diseases. But something more was needed to make sure this broad constituency was heard loud and clear on Capitol Hill.

THIRTEEN

Marching for Progress

—————

As the shadows lengthened across the National Mall near Constitution Avenue, just down the hill from the US Capitol, most of the crowd had dispersed. National Park Service workers moved across the grass picking up "No More Cancer" signs. When they reached a display wall where I sat contemplating, one young man said, "Sir, we're going to have to ask you to move on; we have to disassemble this wall." After some discussion and explanation, he finally agreed to let the wall remain another twenty-four hours.

The wall—a humble monument to children who had succumbed to cancer—was divided into sections for each state. It provided those still grieving an opportunity for some closure. What transfixed me were the poignant remembrances—a favorite toy, a good-bye poem, a pair of tiny sneakers, or a picture of someone cherished—tokens of love for a son, daughter, brother, or sister lost too soon.

Among hundreds of people I greeted that day, September 26, 1998, was a mother who told me she had lost not one, but two daughters to glioblastoma—brain cancer. Treatments had not improved in the years between each child's death. Then she added that the younger daughter had died just within the past week. How could she summon the courage to be here now? "My husband didn't want me to come, but I had to. This is too important. My daughter fought to survive long enough to join the march, but didn't quite make it. So I'm here to represent her."

We called the weekend event "The MARCH: Coming Together to Conquer Cancer." The vice president of the United States and many other prominent speakers filled the program; hundreds of thousands rode buses to Washington and to other cities nationwide. But it was that simple wall that sticks in my memory.

CONSTRUCTING THE MOST EFFECTIVE STRATEGY

That extraordinary event was a key to implementing the strategy of doubling the NIH budget. Momentum began with the 1995 Cancer Summit. Later that year, I delivered a speech in New York attended by Professor Donald Coffey from Johns Hopkins. Don wrote:

Dear Mike,
Your talk was inspiring and moving. We must increase our efforts by orders of magnitude to conquer cancer and we must focus on a *real* war this time . . . We need you to wake up our leaders and to focus government, industry, academia and the public on this scourge until we stamp it out. It will be cured and prevented as the horrors of polio, smallpox and typhoid were defeated—and as AIDS will be too. You said that victory is through research. As the incoming president of the American Association of Can-

cer Research, I pledge my heart and soul to this goal. We will win, as America did in WWII, but it will be a struggle. <u>Let's declare war!</u>

Don Coffey

I assured Don we were planning major new initiatives to step up the pace of our common goal.

Following months of work throughout 1996, we helped achieve passage of the 1997 FDA Modernization Act to fast-track cancer drugs. Also in early 1997, *Larry King Live* featured Ellen Stovall of the NCCS; ABC News commentator and cancer survivor Sam Donaldson; CBS news anchor and breast cancer activist Paula Zahn; talk show host and cancer survivor Morton Downey, Jr.; actor Robert Urich, also a cancer survivor; and me. (Larry had once told me that on the subject of disease, people are more likely to accept the views of celebrities than the pronouncements of doctors.) After each guest had talked about the need for action, Larry asked, "Why don't you form an army of cancer survivors and march on Washington to demand a cure for cancer?"

That challenge from King helped focus the cancer community on the idea of a massive demonstration. A few months later, Stovall, Donaldson, and I returned to *Larry King Live* along with Cindy Crawford, whose brother had died of leukemia; tennis star and children's cancer advocate Andrea Jaeger; and figure skating champion Scott Hamilton, who had survived testicular cancer. We used the opportunity to announce a March on Washington the following September. During the program, General Norman Schwarzkopf, a prostate cancer survivor and hero of the 1991 Gulf War, called in to offer support. He was named honorary chairman of the march.

Schwarzkopf was blunt: "When the American people see how

woefully underfunded cancer research is, they will be mad as hell. I'm going to be at the march and I challenge every other cancer survivor and every other American to be there with me."

Ten key principles for the march then emerged from many long CaP CURE meetings:

1. Build the event around a clear concept everyone can understand. We wanted non-cancer organizations to understand that our efforts to double the NIH budget would advance work on all diseases, thousands of which lacked a cure. But we determined to avoid a fragmented discussion. To bring the message home, the march would focus on cancer, the one disease that puts fear into everyone's hearts and affects virtually every family. This was a central argument of our appeal to Congress.

2. As part of our Capitol Hill education campaign, Intel Chairman Andy Grove and other CaP CURE board members joined me long before the march in calls on more than a hundred members of Congress. After telling them the facts about cancer's impact on their constituents, we noted that a grassroots army of advocates—hundreds of thousands strong—would be coming to Washington and other sites in their home states and districts. It was very much a people's march. We asked them to engage with this "army" and support its objectives. And just so there would be no doubt about their commitment, we recorded interviews with many congressional leaders. When we began to publicize plans for the march, we included recordings of these interviews in the packages sent to local broadcast outlets.

3. The CaP CURE leadership group studied why previous appeals to increase the NIH budget had been largely unsuccessful. The people who made these appeals were intelligent, talented people; yet their pleas had not moved Congress to act. We decided to make the economic argument. Other groups had

limited their appeals to heartrending portrayals of afflicted patients—children in wheelchairs, women who'd lost their hair, or a father hoping to survive long enough to walk his daughter down the aisle. These descriptions can be effective to a point. We went further, backing up the emotional words with cold, hard facts about the cost of failure. Like others, we said every individual life is precious. Then we cited careful analyses by respected economists to show the return on investment in medical research and public health.

4. Recognize that cancer is more than a single disease. It's a constellation of related conditions—at least a hundred of them, many with their own advocacy organizations. Part of our strategy was to create more disease-specific organizations. We told them the goal was to enlarge the financial pie for all disease research, not to shift anyone's slice to another group. Underlying that message were Angus Maddison's famous studies showing that approximately half of all economic growth over the previous two centuries was based on advances in health and longevity.[*]

5. Spread the net far beyond Washington, DC. To reach every corner of America, we recruited organizers for local events hosted at more than fifty NIH-designated Comprehensive Cancer Centers and other important medical institutions in every state. Our message went out to big corporations, mom-and-pop enterprises, labor unions, college students, minority groups, professional associations—everyone who could be affected by cancer (which is to say, everyone). They all had to feel they were part of the event. To that end, we lined up entertainers who would appeal to various demographic groups.

6. Take advantage of leadership by women, not because they are women, but because they had been in the forefront of our successful health-related efforts and broader advocacy programs. Soon after the 1995 Cancer Summit, I met with

---

[*] *Monitoring the World Economy 1820–1992* (OECD, 1995).

the executive director of the National Coalition for Cancer Survivorship (NCCS), Ellen Stovall, who agreed to play a major role in the planning. Other experienced executives who joined the effort were Sherry Lansing, CEO of Paramount Pictures; and Dr. Ellen Sigal, a member of the NCI's Board of Scientific Advisors and chair of Friends of Cancer Research. I asked Dr. Anna Barker, a distinguished scientist with deep knowledge of the federal government's interagency health programs, to develop our research strategy. Among other highly effective women with a targeted focus on specific diseases were Amy Langer, head of the National Alliance of Breast Cancer Organizations, and Fran Visco, an influential lawyer and president of the National Breast Cancer Coalition, a grassroots advocacy organization of more than six hundred member groups and seventy thousand individual members.

7. We stressed that the cancer community should work together rather than pit one organization against another. Like the British colonies represented as pieces of a snake in Benjamin Franklin's famous "Join or Die" cartoon, we needed to play on the same team because that will make us all stronger.*

8. Another strategy was to bring in a large cohort of medical researchers from academic medical centers, government and industry to give our messages additional credibility. We told these physicians and scientists to bring their entire families, especially children, who would see the importance of their life's work. This helped validate their career choices.

---

* American Cancer Society executives didn't like my idea of creating disease-specific organizations. They wanted to be in the forefront, representing all cancer groups. They told me what I was proposing would "fragment the movement." I told them we sought just the opposite—we hoped many of the smaller cancer organizations would merge to improve their efficiency and effectiveness. In the last weeks before the march, the ACS finally recognized the strength of this strategy and joined our team. They helped organize bus trips to Washington by thousands of marchers. Today, the ACS president and CEO is Karen Knudsen, MBA, PhD, a prominent cancer researcher. Dr. Knudsen is a PCF awardee who has participated in our annual scientific retreats. She is the first woman to lead the ACS in its 107-year history.

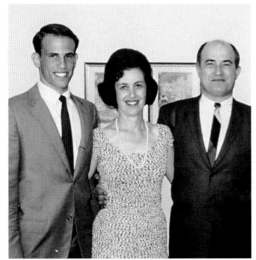

With my parents as a
high school senior.

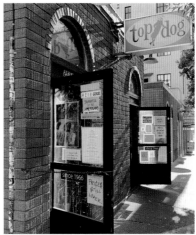

The Top Dog hot dog
shop in Berkeley.

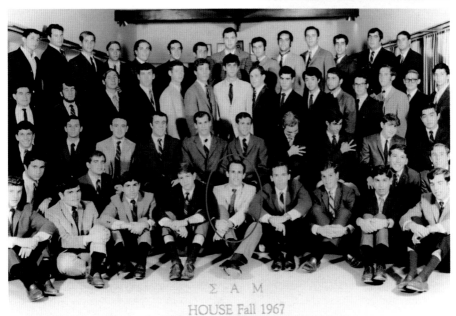

Some of my fraternity brothers at Sigma Alpha Mu in 1967,
when I served as president.

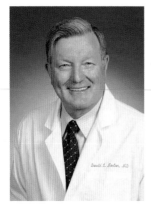
Donald Morton, MD

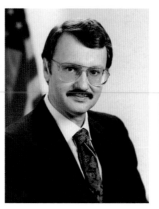
Sam Broder, MD

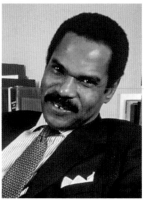
Reginald Lewis

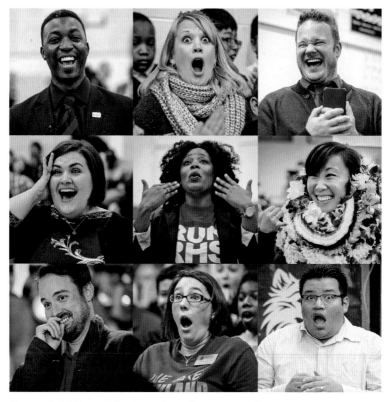

Stunned Milken Educator Award winners, above, react to surprise announcements of their selections. Some three thousand Milken Educators since the 1980s have inspired millions of students, many of whom pursued careers in medicine, health and science. See www.fastercurebook .com.

These four cancer leaders were the nucleus of my original treatment team in 1993.

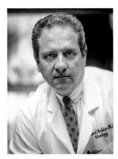 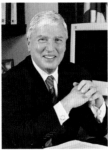 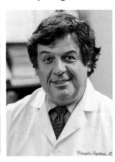 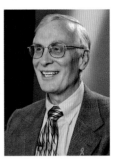

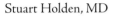

Stuart Holden, MD

Andrew von Eschenbach, MD

Christopher Logothetis, MD

Charles Myers, MD

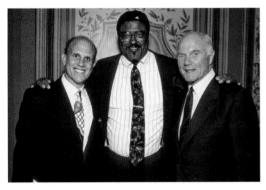

The Reverend Rosey Grier, shown here with the late senator John Glenn and me in 1993, was known as an imposing presence on the football field, yet the "Gentle Giant" later inspired congregations from the pulpit and helped lead CaP CURE programs.

2010 PCF Young Investigator Himisha Beltran, MD, a medical oncologist at Harvard's Dana Farber Cancer Institute, now mentors other early-career scientists.

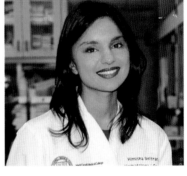

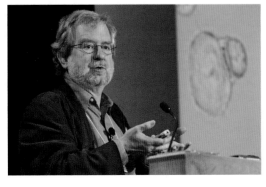

Dr. James Allison at an early CaP CURE Scientific Retreat many years before he won the Nobel Prize.

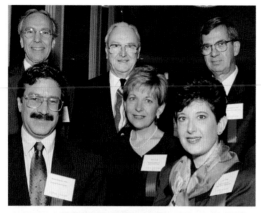

Richard Klausner, MD, then-director of the National Cancer Institute (*front left*) was joined at the National Cancer Summit by former NCI directors (*back row*) Arthur Upton, MD, Carl Baker, MD, and Vincent DeVita Jr., MD, as well as Ellen Stovall, executive director of the National Coalition for Cancer Survivorship and Amy Langer of the Breast Cancer Alliance (*right*).

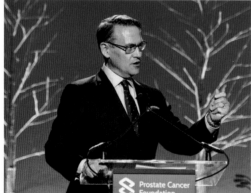

Charles (Chuck) Ryan, MD, PCF president and CEO

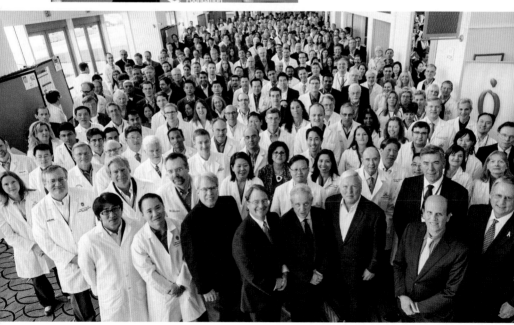

Some of our Young Investigators

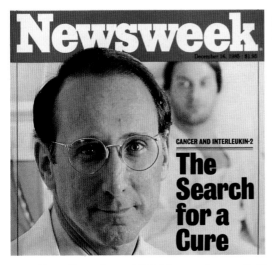
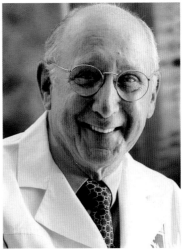

Steve Rosenberg: 1985 *Newsweek* cover (*left*); Steve in a recent photo (*right*)

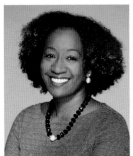
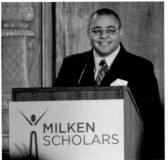
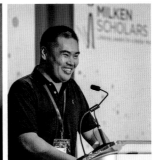

Lori and I developed the Milken Scholars program to encourage outstanding high school seniors from low socioeconomic levels who have excelled in academic performance, community service, leadership, and ability to overcome obstacles. Many have become physicians and scientists. Left to right: Joelle Simpson, MD; Henry Horton, MD; and John Shen, MD. See www.fastercuresbook.com.

A *Forbes* magazine cover story highlighted programs of the Milken Scholars and the Milken Educator Awards.

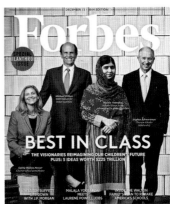

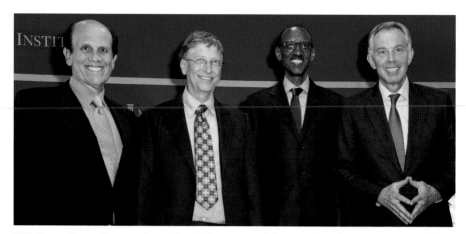

Bill Gates, Rwandan president Paul Kagame, and former British prime minister Tony Blair joined me on a 2013 Milken Institute Global Conference panel to discuss progress and challenges in providing comprehensive health services in Africa.

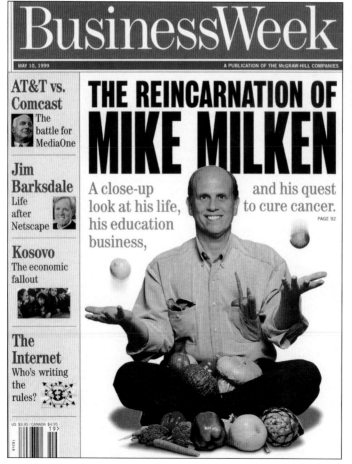

One of many articles that promoted nutrition.

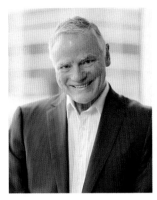
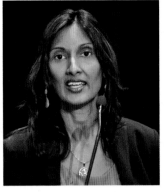
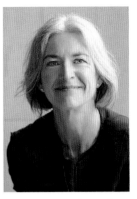

Lee Hood, MD, PhD   Padmanee (Pam) Sharma,   Jennifer Doudna, PhD
                        MD, PhD

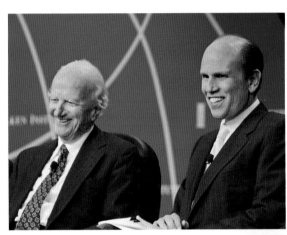

Gary Becker often joined me on conference panels.

Vice President Al Gore at the 1998 March on Washington: "We want to be the generation that wins the war on cancer."

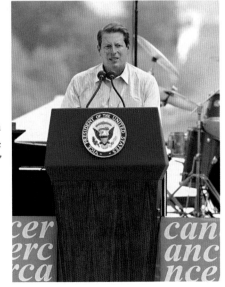

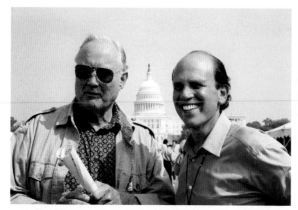

General Norman Schwarzkopf joined me at the March.

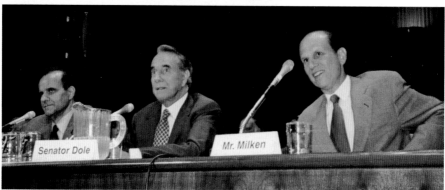

Joe Torre, Bob Dole, and I testified before a Senate subcommittee in 1999.

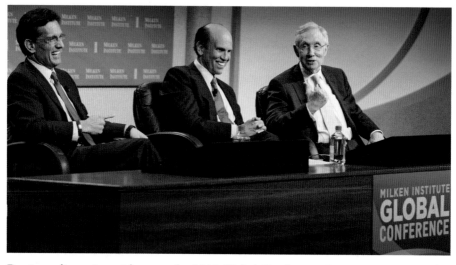

During a discussion with me at the 2013 Global Conference, House Majority Leader Eric Cantor, a Republican, and Senate Majority Leader Harry Reid, a Democrat, acknowledged that they should spend more time fostering bipartisan relations.

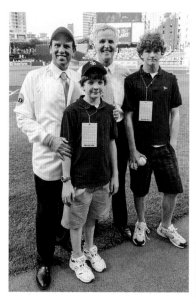

Trip Casscells with his sons, Henry and Sam, joined me at Baltimore's Oriole Park at Camden Yards for a Home Run Challenge game.

Trip, on my right, and Larry Stupski at Lake Tahoe late in their struggles against prostate cancer. Larry was the former president and CEO of Charles Schwab Corporation and a visionary philanthropist. Trip and Larry both served on the PCF board of directors.

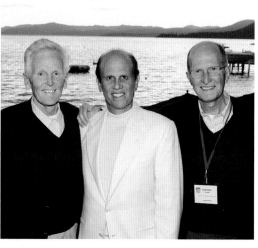

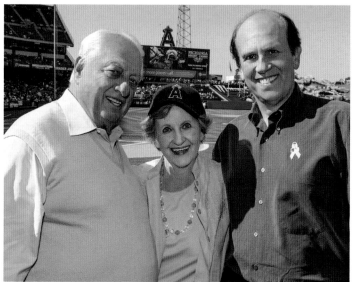

Dodgers legend the late Tommy Lasorda, with my mother and me at a Home Run Challenge game.

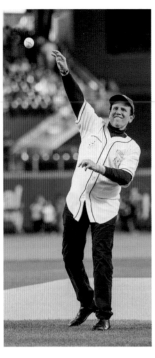

After throwing the first pitch at a Major League Baseball game, I decided to keep my day job.

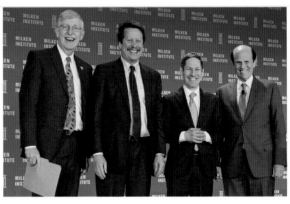

NIH Director Francis Collins, FDA Commissioner Robert Califf, and CDC Director Tom Frieden spoke at a *FasterCures* Future of Health Summit.

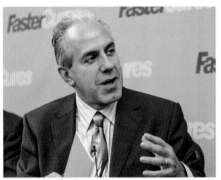

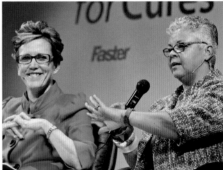

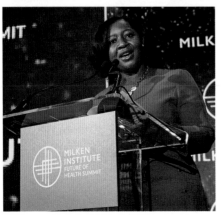

Greg Simon (*above left*), the first executive director of *FasterCures*, was succeeded by Margaret Anderson (*above right, in blue dress*). Dr. Freda Lewis-Hall joined Margaret on a Partnering for Cures panel. *FasterCures* was later headed by Esther Krofah (*left*), who led its responses to the COVID-19 crisis.

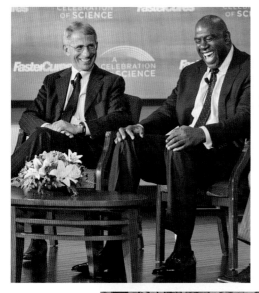

Dr. Tony Fauci with Magic Johnson.

Some of the Rock Docs backstage at the Kennedy Center.

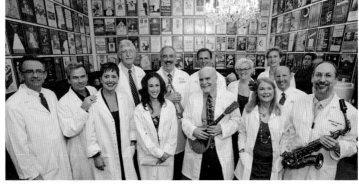

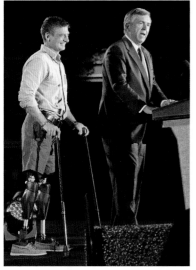

At the Celebration of Science, Captain Dan Berschinski (USA, Ret.) joins General Peter Chiarelli (USA, Ret.) to report on advances in treating wounded warriors.

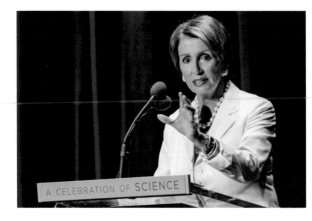

House Speaker Nancy Pelosi at the Celebration of Science.

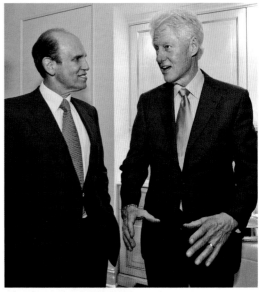

Former president Bill Clinton met with me following a 2011 New York event to raise funds for medical research. The next year, he spoke at the Milken Institute Global Conference. During his administration, he signed legislation that doubled the NIH budget and speeded access to cancer drugs.

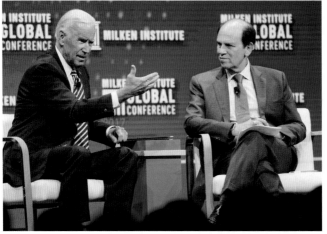

President Joe Biden, who lost a son to cancer, discussed his commitment to medical research at the twentieth annual Milken Institute Global Conference.

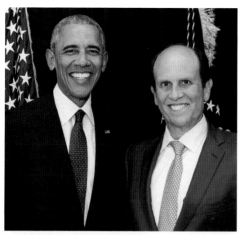

At the White House with President Barack Obama, who had signed the Act creating NCATS and, later, the 21st Century Cures Act.

Below: President George W. Bush told a Global Conference audience about the PEPFAR program funding HIV treatments in Africa.

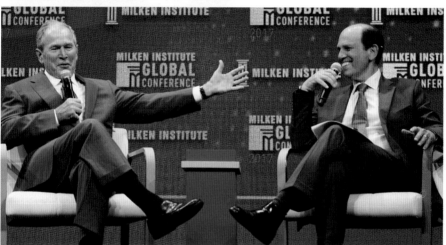

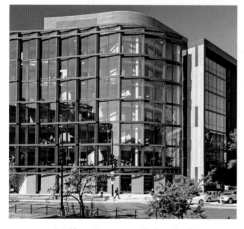

Milken Institute School of Public Health (MISPH)

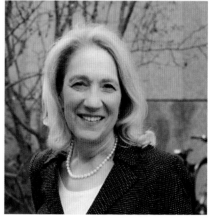

Lynn Goldman, MD, MPH, Dean of the MISPH

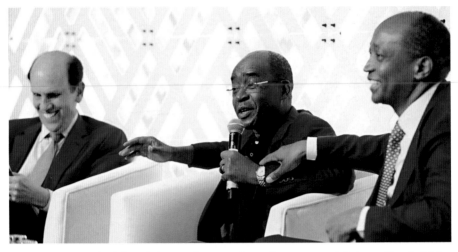

Patrice Motespe (*right*) and Strive Masiyiwa (*center*) join me in 2020 at a South Africa medical conference for alumni Scholars of the International Finance Corporation-Milken Institute (IFC-MI) Capital Markets Program. The IFC, part of the World Bank Group, partners with us to bring mid-career finance professionals to George Washington University for a one-year academic/internship program.

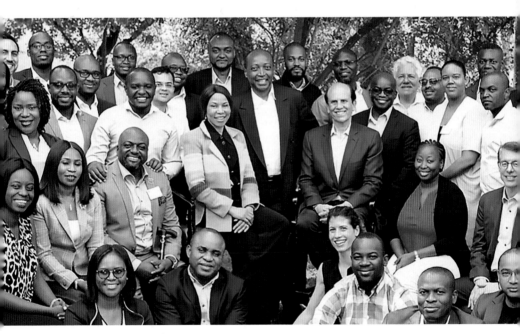

Patrice and Precious Motsepe (*center, to my right*) with some of IFC-MI Scholars at the South Africa medical conference. These Scholars are changing the lives of millions by helping develop greater prosperity in the developing world . . . and with it, improved health.

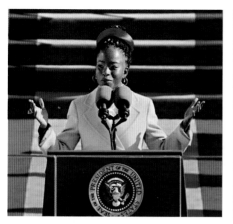
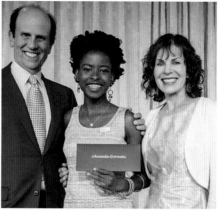

Milken Scholar Amanda Gorman reading her poem "The Hill We Climb" at the January 2021 Presidential Inauguration. Four years earlier, Lori and I presented Amanda with her Scholar award as she prepared to enter Harvard.

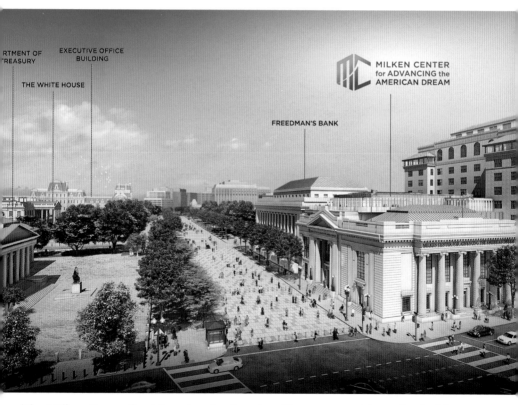

The Milken Center for Advancing the American Dream, comprising a five-building campus connected by an enclosed atrium, is across the street from the Treasury and the White House on historic Pennsylvania Avenue.

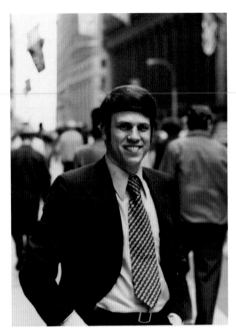

Outside my New York office, 1973.

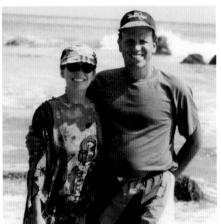

With Lori at the beach, 1993.

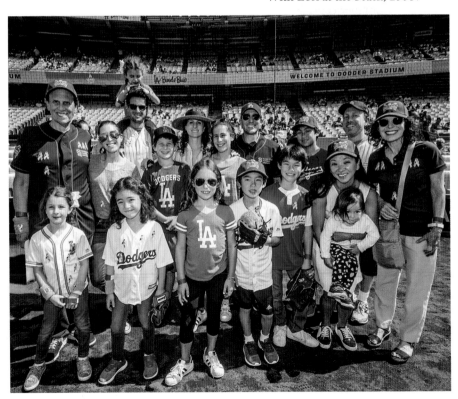

With Lori and our three children, their spouses, and our ten grandchildren.

9. We asked hundreds of groups to join us and told them they would not have to pay to participate. We'd raise the necessary funds and give them an equal seat at the table because we wanted their ideas and commitment. We gave each organization its own booth on the National Mall and encouraged them to pitch in. Eventually, six hundred groups signed on and helped us mobilize half a million people nationwide for a coordinated and effective effort. Estimates of the cost ranged up to ten million dollars. The situation reminded me of 1993, when we kick-started the growth of prostate cancer research with a $25 million grant from the Milken Family Foundation rather than wait until enough smaller contributions had been collected. During the planning for the March, I persuaded Sidney Kimmel, founder and chairman of the Jones Apparel Group and a longtime medical philanthropist, to join me in committing $5 million each. Smaller contributions came in later.

10. A final strategy involved communications. I spoke about our plans in dozens of speeches around the country. In those days before the rise of social media, we made extensive use of radio and television.

The thread tying all these strategies together was inclusivity. During the months leading up to the march, we recruited the "army." With the growing use of the internet, word quickly spread across the country that something very important was soon going to happen on the National Mall.

FINAL PREPARATIONS

Early in July 1998, breast cancer survivor Dani Grady of San Diego started Conquer Cancer Coast to Coast, an eleven-week, 3,600-mile bicycle ride across the US. Joined by other riders along the way, Grady planned to lead the group onto the Mall during the march. Other activists helped organize local rallies, marches, town hall meetings, and vigils in cities nationwide. Governors and mayors issued proclamations.

On July 15, a large, CaP CURE–sponsored van pulled up to the east front of the US Capitol to offer prostate and breast cancer screenings for members of Congress. Aside from the public service of the screenings, it turned out to be an effective way to raise our profile and preview the march. As luck would have it, a rare joint session of Congress was held that day to hear a speech by a visiting head of state. Most members of Congress and many of their spouses attended, assuring a steady flow of visitors to the van.

Near the VIP entrance to the Capitol stood CaP CURE board member Rosey Grier, an imposing six-foot-five-inch former member of the Los Angeles Rams' Fearsome Foursome, one of the greatest defensive lines in football history. Despite an appearance that many would find intimidating, Rosey was known as a friendly "gentle giant." With utmost courtesy, Rosey told visitors they should be tested in our van before entering the Capitol. When Emil Constantinescu, the president of Romania, approached with his entourage, Rosey shocked His Excellency by suggesting he get a prostate test. I guess when you've sacked the greatest quarterbacks in football, no foreign official fazes you. But this had the makings of an international incident. Breaking the tension, Representative Maxine Waters, who had just received a mammogram, intervened and suggested a compromise: The president would be most welcome inside the Capitol if one of his senior staff agreed to be tested. Incident defused.

AN INEXTINGUISHABLE CANDLE

Beginning on September 25, marchers across the eastern half of the United States piled onto buses bound for Washington. (One devoted busload of women from Alabama traveled fourteen hours nonstop, attended the march the next day, then turned around to go home.)

Early that Friday evening, Vice President Al Gore and his wife, Tipper, held a reception for several hundred march organizers and participants. We met in a tent on the grounds of the Naval Observatory, the vice presidential residence. Gore invited a few of us into the residence to discuss the event and soon agreed to speak the next day.

Later, as the sun eased below the western end of the Mall, tens of thousands of cancer survivors gathered at the Lincoln Memorial for a candlelight vigil to honor the memory of those who had lost their lives to cancer. After an interfaith service, General Schwarzkopf, Scott Hamilton, Andrea Jaeger, and other celebrities made brief speeches. Following a musical performance, the Reverend Jesse Jackson rose to speak. He began softly, then gradually raised his booming voice to exhort the gathering:

> *We will out-dream, out-work, out-research, out-fight! We will conquer cancer because our minds are made up. Tonight we march for public policy, new priorities; we march for our basic rights, the right to live, the right to breathe, the right to build, the right to grow, the right to family.*

As people stood holding candles, one woman said she was a survivor of more than ten reoccurrences of cancer, but she was "a candle that cannot be extinguished." It's hard to imagine the courage it takes to endure all those treatments.

NO MORE CANCER

On Saturday, the Mall was dotted with white tents housing cancer education and prevention displays. In one tent, several of the speakers and performers autographed a poster commemorating the march. The signers included former US senator and presidential nominee Bob Dole; and recording artist Graham Nash of the group Crosby, Stills & Nash.

It was an ironic pairing: In 1969, a young and conservative Robert Dole from Kansas was giving his maiden speech in the US Senate, the ultimate bastion of American tradition. That same year, Graham Nash, with defiant long hair, was performing at Woodstock before a crowd of half-dressed young people bent on strengthening a counterculture opposed to the establishment Dole represented. Dole had won two Purple Hearts in World War II; the Woodstock crowd vehemently opposed the Vietnam War. But on the Mall, Nash said to me, "I never thought I'd be in such agreement with Senator Dole, much less signing the same document."

King Hussein of Jordan, who would lose his life to cancer just a few months later, had flown in that day against the advice of his doctors, who were treating him at the Mayo Clinic. He planned to speak but was too weak to do so. His wife, Queen Noor, took his place and made an emotional appeal.

As the formal program began under a baking midday sun, Vice President Gore tossed his suit jacket aside, rolled up his sleeves, and told the crowd, "Some people still say it is impossible to find a cancer cure. A hundred years ago, people said the same thing about smallpox."

Speaker after speaker—Schwarzkopf, Tipper Gore, Queen Noor, Senator Connie Mack, Sidney Kimmel, ABC political analyst Cokie Roberts, Sam Donaldson, and several more—were greeted with enthusiastic cheers. After Aretha Franklin electrified the audience with some gospel and soul standards, she wrote a check to help with the march expenses.

Then it was my turn. "My name is Mike Milken and I am a cancer survivor." The crowd yelled encouragement. "You make history today," I continued.

Today we are united to defeat cancer. Today in Washington we think back to our parents, our grandparents and generations of Americans who fought to make this country free and give us a better life. We think back to generations of Americans and scientists who have rid us of smallpox and polio. My father had polio but he died from cancer. It's our commitment today that our children will not remember cancer. For those children and the children of future generations, let's get on with finding a cure for cancer and let's do it now.

After pedaling across the Mall—the last lap of her cross-country ride—an excited Dani Grady bounded up the steps of the speakers' platform hoisting her bicycle over her head. "I've been waiting a long time to say this—Hello Washington! Hello America!" Then, echoing Henry V before the battle of Agincourt, she added, "Remember where you were today."

Sprinkled among the crowd were many cancer scientists and physicians who had never seen this kind of mass rally. Dr. Jonathan Simons, then at Johns Hopkins and later head of the Prostate Cancer Foundation, brought his wife and told his two young sons this is why he went into medicine. Dr. Joel Nelson, a prominent urologist, brought his entire family and later wrote:

It's not often that you're involved in something with this kind of magnitude. As a doctor who cares for cancer patients, I was really inspired. It made me think of what we're capable of. All that stands between us and success is our saying, "Let's get going."

LONG-TERM IMPACT OF THE MARCH

Our ten-point strategy worked. The strength of our numbers, the unity and commitment of hundreds of individuals and organizations, and the years we'd spent calling on members of Congress—it all came together to change the history of disease research. There was still much work to do, but the march was a turning point, the culmination of CaP CURE's first five years. Within a month, President Clinton signed the first of several bills that would eventually double the NIH budget.

As part of our efforts to maintain the momentum of the march, we hosted a meeting at Lake Tahoe for several major funders of cancer research—the National Cancer Institute, the Department of Defense, the American Cancer Society, CaP CURE, and others. This led to a Funders Conference in Washington attended by Richard Klausner, then the NCI Director; Andy Grove; government officials from other agencies; and business executives representing major health sciences companies. That meeting and similar conferences over the next several years helped refine the NCI's cancer strategy.

The following summer, I was invited to testify about cancer funding before the US Senate Subcommittee on Labor, Health and Human Services, and Education Appropriations. I asked Joe Torre, the manager of the New York Yankees, who had recently been diagnosed with prostate cancer, if he'd also like to make a statement to the committee. It was June, the middle of baseball season, and

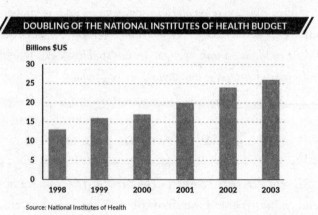

DOUBLING OF THE NATIONAL INSTITUTES OF HEALTH BUDGET

Billions $US

Source: National Institutes of Health

Torre couldn't be away from the team for long. I agreed to pick him up in the morning at his suburban New York home and fly with him to Washington, getting us back to Yankee Stadium for that night's game. On the outbound flight, I reviewed prepared remarks with a colleague: "I don't think these numbers are right. You see here where it compares cancer funding to the gross domestic product? There should be another zero before the decimal point."

Torre, chewing on a bagel across the aisle, turned to me: "Geez, Mike, I don't know about those numbers. All I know about math is if I have more than nine guys on the field, I'm f—ed!" Later that day, Bob Dole sat with Joe and me as the three of us testified before the committee. I reminded the senators about the previous year's march:

> *How much firepower do we need to defeat cancer? Last fall, as part of The March, we suggested that the annual federal investment in cancer research be increased to $10 billion. That's less than forty dollars per American. It is a fraction of the cost of failure—the cost of treating more than a hundred million Americans currently living who are expected to get cancer.*
>
> *I believe we can accelerate science. If we give cancer researchers the same kinds of tools that technology companies employ in accelerating scientific development, we can find a cure faster . . . Let's send a message to our brightest young scientists that cancer research is an exciting profession. Finally, let's show all these dedicated people that we share their sense of urgency.*

The higher base of NIH funding that President Clinton signed into law has meant hundreds of billions of dollars more for lifesaving research in the years since. No one will ever know exactly how many lives that increase saved, but no doubt the research it enabled has brought us closer to important medical solutions—to faster cures.

GETTING TO ZERO DEATHS

While the broad impacts of the NIH budget increase are difficult to measure with precision, we do have some data. We know, for example, that there are 3.7 million more cancer survivors than was predicted when we launched CaP CURE in 1993. Ten years after that 1993 launch, the celebrated Johns Hopkins surgeon, Patrick Walsh, wrote:

> *All of a sudden, there was opportunity with a relatively simple, rapid-review process to apply for funding. So young investigators without a track record, who would have had difficulty receiving government grants, were able to get pilot projects funded. These individuals solidified their careers in this field because of the opportunity for funding, and then, once the government caught on, were able to get continued grants. History will show that cancer research bloomed when CaP CURE began. They've done more than any other organization to reduce deaths.*

In 2020, management consultants McKinsey & Company put specific numbers on that assessment. They studied several disease foundations to see how well they spent their budgets. Their report showed that for every $10 million of research dollars spent, the Prostate Cancer Foundation (CaP CURE's successor) prevented 815 deaths per 100,000 men. Looking at comparable populations for different disease groups, the next most efficient foundation (the Milken Institute-affiliated Melanoma Research Alliance) saved 546 lives. For the third group listed, it was 303 lives saved. In other words, the PCF saved almost as many lives as the next two foundations combined.*

---

* The McKinsey report estimated that the PCF could reduce deaths from prostate cancer to zero by 2051 at its current funding level assuming incremental development without a

Analyzing how CaP CURE and the PCF achieved these remarkable results, McKinsey pointed to several medical milestones in which we were directly involved. (Nontechnical readers will find explanations of some words in the following list at www.pcf.org.)

- 1996: Discovery of inherited genes in familial prostate cancer (PC).

- 1999: The first liquid biopsy science conference.

- 2000: Approval of the first robotic surgery system for PC.

- 2004: Approval of docetaxel for metastatic castration-resistant prostate cancer (mCRPC).

- 2007: Image-guided radiation therapy (IGRT) becomes standard of care.

- 2010: Sipuleucel-T becomes first immunotherapy for PC.

- 2010: Approval of cabazitaxel for mCRPC.

- 2011: Approval of abiraterone for mCRPC.

- 2012: Approval of enzalutamide for mCRPC.

- 2013: Approval of radium-223 for mCRPC.

- 2015: Docetaxel for metastatic hormone-sensitive prostate cancer (mHSPC).

- 2015: Discovery of inherited DNA repair mutations that drive PC.

- 2017: Approval of pembrolizumab for hyper-mutated cancers.

- 2020: Olaparib and rucaparib for BRCA 1/2 mutant mCRPC.

---

major success in its priority research areas. The report further estimated that zero deaths could be achieved by 2038 if the foundation could double its investment in research. A best-case assumption in the report said that a major breakthrough in one or more of twenty priority pipeline areas could bring eradication as soon as 2031.

In 2022, the FDA followed up on the 2015 approval of docetaxel for mHSPC by adding its approval of darolutamide, which creates an enhanced option for patients whose cancer has spread beyond the prostate.

THE GIRL FROM GUYANA

Doubling of the NIH budget was an investment of billions in research that created trillions of dollars' worth of human capital over the years. The specific impact becomes clearer if we look at some of the medical scientists whose crucial work was funded as part of the larger NIH budget. One of them is Pam Sharma.

Padmanee (Pam) Sharma, MD, PhD, today is a professor in the Department of Immunology at the MD Anderson Cancer Center in Houston. A leading figure in oncology, her primary focus is on the immune system's mechanisms for rejecting tumors. Earlier in her career, she received one of our Young Investigator Awards when she was at Memorial Sloan Kettering Cancer Center in New York. After that, her career blossomed, and she's since received numerous awards for her lifesaving work. Recently, Pam was inducted into the American Society for Clinical Investigation (ASCI). You'd be forgiven for assuming she had a smooth path to such a distinguished career. That's not quite how it happened.

Pam's great-great-grandparents, indentured laborers from India, were sold into slavery during the nineteenth-century British Raj.* In a sense, they were the lucky ones—many died on the boat trip from India to the sugar plantations of Guyana on the northern coast of

---

* Technically, Britain had outlawed slavery. But a brisk trade continued in "indentured laborers" who were shipped to British colonies around the world where they were brutally exploited under contracts specifying wages of pennies a day.

South America. Her grandmother was not allowed to go to school and was married off as a young teenager. So poor that she needed to cook the same chicken bones over and over, she constantly told her fourteen children about the importance of education.

When Pam was seven, she was seriously injured in an accident and lay in a coma for weeks. Upon awakening, she was so impressed by the doctors who cared for her she decided to go to medical school, an unheard-of aspiration for a Guyanese girl. By good fortune, her parents immigrated to "Little Guyana" in Queens, New York. Some immigrants never look back, but Pam didn't forget the plight of girls in Guyana. During her medical training, she returned to her homeland and started a foundation to encourage the educational advancement of young girls. That foundation got a big boost when her husband, James Allison, won the $3 million Breakthrough Prize in Life Sciences in 2014 and then the 2018 Nobel Prize in Medicine. The couple decided to donate the prize money to Pam's foundation.

FOURTEEN

Home Runs for Cures

As we inched along through bumper-to-bumper traffic, it seemed as if every car in Chicago was headed to the same destination: historic Wrigley Field. Tommy Lasorda, the great former manager of the Los Angeles Dodgers and member of baseball's Hall of Fame, sat next to me. Our chances of snagging a parking space near the main entry were slim, but we decided to give it a try.

"You can't park there!" shouted a security guard when we approached the famous entrance. Then he recognized Tommy, asked for an autograph, and suddenly found us a parking space. Ernie Banks, the former Chicago Cubs Hall of Fame player known as "Mr. Cub," came out to greet us. We were there as representatives of CaP CURE for the Home Run Challenge (HRC), our national fundraising and awareness promotion with Major League Baseball. The memorable game that afternoon made the day—June 7, 2003—very special.

No one needed an explanation of the three-word message on the stadium's iconic marquee: "Wood vs. Clemens." A standing-room-only crowd of nearly forty thousand was buzzing about the matchup between the New York Yankees' six-time Cy Young Award winner, Roger Clemens, looking for his three hundredth career win, and twenty-five-year-old Cubs phenom, Kerry Wood, who led the majors in strikeouts.

It was also the first Yankees' appearance at the fabled North Side ballpark since they'd swept the 1938 World Series. Walking onto that same field, I looked at the ivy-covered outfield wall, inhaled the aromas, and listened to the shouts of the peanut, beer, and hot dog vendors.

This must have been what it was like in 1938.

Before the game, I chatted with Cubs manager Dusty Baker, a prostate cancer survivor and strong HRC supporter. Surely his lineup card would include Eric Karros, who had hit the most home runs in our HRC games over the past several years. Dusty told me Karros wasn't in the opening lineup—he wanted a left-hander at first base to face Clemens.

What? No Karros? I told Dusty he was making a mistake, but he didn't agree.

Clemens was at the top of his game as he attempted to win number three hundred. Wood was hoping to win his fiftieth. At one point, Clemens retired fifteen consecutive batters. Yet the younger Wood matched him pitch for pitch, carrying a no-hitter through several innings.

In a near-tragic fourth-inning moment, Wood collided with starting first baseman Hee-seop Choi as they both ran to catch a pop fly that was blown off course by the wind whipping off Lake Michigan. Choi made the catch, but took the brunt of the collision and lay unconscious while an ambulance emerged from under the stands. With

Choi headed to the hospital, Baker pointed toward the dugout and called for Karros to play first base.

By the sixth inning, the forty-year-old Clemens began to tire. Clinging to a 1–0 lead, he allowed two runners to reach base in the bottom of the seventh. Yankees manager Joe Torre, also a prostate cancer survivor, brought in reliever Juan Acevedo. If the lead held, Clemens would have his three hundredth victory.

Next up was Karros. Acevedo grimaced and shook his head, calling off two signs from the catcher. Then he let loose with a high fastball. The crack of the bat could be heard out on Sheffield Avenue as Karros smacked a towering home run over the left-field bleachers. "The stadium was out of control," Wood said. "You couldn't hear yourself think. It was awesome." Wood held the Yanks at bay into the eighth inning and came away with a 5–2 victory. It was one of the greatest games in Chicago sports history.

THE AMERICAN PASTIME

The idea for the Home Run Challenge that brought us to the Windy City that day began many years earlier during a brainstorming session at our Santa Monica headquarters. We wanted to develop creative programs that would raise funds for medical research and increase public awareness of available cancer tests. The 1995 National Cancer Summit in Washington had filled us with optimism about progress against cancer. What tempered that optimism was the discouraging fact that so many men weren't getting a simple, inexpensive screening test. I would not have been there had it not been for my insistence on having my PSA checked a few years earlier.

Think about what you would do if you needed a plan to convince millions of people to take some action that they're inclined to put off—something like seeing a doctor. We needed a way to deliver the message without lecturing, to make it fun and entertaining. Sitting in our third-floor conference room, Rosey Grier and I debated many ideas. As a former professional football player, it was natural for Rosey to suggest a tie-in to sports. But what sport? The pace of basketball and hockey seemed too fast to allow our full messages to get through. Football had longer breaks, but was played only once a week, sometimes in rain or even snow.

Then, as I gazed out the window, I had an inspiration. Our offices were in a modern building only four blocks from the Pacific Ocean. The south, east, and west windows offered appealing views of water and mountains. The north-facing offices, however, looked out on the ugly concrete-block side of a parking garage owned by the City of Santa Monica. After receiving permission from the city, we commissioned an artist to cover the garage wall with a huge mural depicting colorful scenes of the area's history. Now the view from the conference room window showed happy beachgoers playing in the sunshine. This piece of public art helped bring the outside in for some of our employees.

That's when it occurred to me that baseball, the "great American pastime," was a popular sport that's usually played in the healthy outdoors. Many of us have pleasant childhood memories of going to a ballgame with our fathers and grandfathers, the exact audience we needed to reach.

The pace of baseball offered plenty of opportunities to talk between plays. But we needed an exciting way to link our messages to the game and to raise funds for research. What's the most exciting play in baseball? The home run! Maybe we could link the promotion to home runs and center it around Father's Day, which falls in the middle of baseball season. Baseball, home runs, Father's Day—it seemed like a great combination.

Over the next few months, we developed the concept in a series of planning sessions. We'd ask for contributions linked to the number of home runs hit in specified Major League games during the weeks leading up to Father's Day. Our slogan would be "Keep Dad in the Game." The next challenge was to sell it to the owners of Major League Baseball teams.

During the annual winter meeting of all the owners, I arranged a private breakfast with three of them—Peter Magowan of the San Francisco Giants, Jerry Reinsdorf of the Chicago White Sox, and Fred Wilpon of the New York Mets—whom I knew from my business career. If I could convince them that an MLB-CaP CURE partnership would be good for baseball, maybe they'd pitch the idea to the other owners. I explained that our promotion would involve everyone connected to the sport including players, coaches, fans, broadcasters—even umpires and groundskeepers—as well as owners. It would help save lives and portray the teams as public-spirited organizations.

My breakfast guests asked lots of questions. One concern was that the subject of cancer would be a downer just when they were searching for new ways to show fans and spectators a good time. We all agreed that many men are reluctant to see their doctors for what could be a lifesaving blood test. So I brought up the idea that baseball stars could be effective role models and spokesmen. Eventually, the three owners came around and said they'd recommend a promotional partnership to the other owners.

TREASURED MEMORIES

The MLB owners not only approved what became the Home Run Challenge—they backed it enthusiastically and have continued to do so for more than a quarter century. Our HRC team has been to more than five hundred games in all thirty ballparks. Each year, I participate at stadiums around the country, sometimes getting to two cities in a day. By flying west to pick up extra hours, we once even squeezed in three games in a day.

Over the years, the HRC has become one of the world's leading prostate cancer fundraising and awareness campaigns. More than a hundred All-Stars and active ballplayers have hit nearly five thousand home runs during HRC games. Dozens of Hall of Fame members have joined our team over the years including Willie Mays, Frank Robinson, Ernie Banks, Dennis Eckersley, Reggie Jackson, and Derek Jeter.

Late in his life, "Mr. Cardinal," the legendary St. Louis Cardinals slugger Stan Musial, joined me before a Home Run Challenge game at a local Sam's Club. "Stan the Man" was gracious in giving autographs and helping me sign copies of our *Taste for Living* cookbooks, which raised money for cancer research.

Many other stars have pitched in for the cause including Joe Torre when he was manager of the Yankees. At my recommendation, he drank a daily soy shake that's featured in one of our healthy eating cookbooks. But it's where and when he drank it that was so helpful. As the Yankee Stadium organist played "Take Me Out to the Ball Game" during the seventh-inning stretch of home games, Joe appeared on the dugout steps and hoisted his glass for all to see.

TOMMY

Of all the luminaries who traveled with us over the years, there's a special place in my heart for baseball's greatest ambassador, Tommy Lasorda. Tommy passed away before I wrote this, but he will never fade from my memory. He was with us every year from 1997 through 2020, longer than his Hall of Fame career managing his beloved Los Angeles Dodgers.

The stories about Tommy are endless. One day, we attended a Capitol Hill ceremony with several US senators. It was an uncomfortably hot and humid late spring day and we wore lightweight clothes. Later that afternoon, we flew north to Boston for an HRC night game at Fenway Park. The game-time temperature fell into the forties, and everyone in our group gladly accepted bright red warm-up jackets emblazoned with the Red Sox logo. Everyone except Tommy. "I'd rather freeze than wear anything but Dodger blue" was his teeth-chattering response.

At one Yankee Stadium game, several of New York's finest on the security detail lined up to get Tommy's autograph. Grinning ear to ear, the Los Angeles–based Lasorda complimented "the second-best police force in America" as he signed their programs and jerseys.

One night in Cincinnati, Mr. Red, the team's mascot, rushed up to embrace me. Atop the baseball that served as the head of his costume was a large baseball cap. The rock-hard plastic brim of the cap collided with my head and nearly knocked me out. Tommy chased the poor guy around the field yelling some unprintable words in Spanish.

We had a lot of fun and I miss Tommy every day. He was always entertaining. More importantly, his sheer humanity shone through in everything he did.

GETTING INVOLVED

Since 1996, my role in the Home Run Challenge has often included a pregame appearance at home plate to encourage contributions from fans, sometimes displaying an oversized check showing a team donation. Then I go to the broadcast booth to talk about what viewers' contributions have produced in terms of advanced therapies. This is also an opportunity to discuss good nutrition, which can help prevent cancer or slow its growth. And when I'm on the air, I never miss a chance to stress the importance of getting tested. Many people have told me they were checked as a result. Those tests save lives.

The HRC has raised more than $70 million over the years. When you combine that with all the other PCF fundraising programs, we've brought in more than $1 billion. No other program has done more to bring the facts about prostate cancer to men and their families.

Among many personal HRC memories are the time a broadcast producer suggested I operate one of the television cameras for an inning. How hard could that be? You just look through the lens and follow the ball, right? It turns out to be a tricky job best left to the technical professionals. Trying to track a high fly to center field, I swung the camera wildly and completely lost sight of the ball. Then there was the time during a pregame warm-up at Boston's Fenway Park when I decided to shag some balls bouncing off the left-field fence—the "Green Monster." Soon baseballs were flying everywhere—off the hitting-practice bats, on the wall behind me, thrown between outfielders. One of the coaches said, "Who is that guy? He's going to get killed."

I've even thrown out the ceremonial first pitch at several games. (It's always fun to do this and it's for a good cause, but no team has offered me a pitching contract. Two of my grandsons have carried on the tradition, throwing out the first pitch at Giants, Dodgers, and Diamondbacks games.) This isn't to honor us, however. The honors are for the medical scientists whose breakthroughs against cancer are extending the lives of patients everywhere. The appearances are only to draw attention to their achievements so fans will support them.

My Little League playmates from the 1950s must be surprised because back then I was mainly an outfielder who never tried pitching. These days, I usually manage to get the ball to the same zip code as home plate without making a fool of myself. Houston's Minute Maid Park is one of the stadiums where I've done this several times.

HOW MUCH IS A LIFE WORTH?

Houston is where I first met Trip Casscells when he attended an Astros game with his two sons. Astros owner Drayton McLane had invited Trip and the boys to join me in his owner's box after my pre-game ceremonies on the field. Trip is more than a profile in courage—he's a testament to the progress of medical science since the mid-twentieth century.

Samuel Ward Casscells III, MD, known to his friends as "Trip," was chief of cardiology at the University of Texas Medical School. When I met him in 2001 , he was a doctor of considerable renown who'd been consulted by both presidents Bush. One night, Trip woke with pain in his abdomen, where he discovered a lump. His doctor sent him for an MRI. A young radiologist looking at his scan, and unaware that Trip hadn't yet received a diagnosis, casually said, "Gee, there are a lot of metastases here. What's your primary cancer?"

"I just remember my blood turning to ice," said Trip. A blood test and biopsy confirmed a very aggressive form of prostate cancer that had spread throughout his body. Only forty-eight, his life expectancy was three months to a year. "I wanted to scream or cry, but I didn't have time. I envisioned writing letters to my children for them to remember me. It was overwhelming." Trip and his wife, Roxanne, consulted two of the same doctors who had been on my treatment team eight years earlier: Chris Logothetis and Andy von Eschenbach. Chris offered some hope by saying "We'll get you fixed up" and by prescribing a new treatment program developed with PCF funding.

Trip compiled a long list of things to accomplish in his remaining time. He returned to medical practice, published articles, joined the PCF board, led efforts to help Hurricane Katrina victims, patented new medical devices, wrote a book, traveled to Asia to assist victims of an Indonesian tsunami, and aided Pakistani earthquake survivors.

That was just the beginning. Sometime after Trip and I became friends, he mentioned he was about to join the army. What? He told me he was "filled with shame" when his eight-year-old son asked, "Daddy, what did you do during the Vietnam War?" Even though he'd been in medical school during that war training for a career that would save an untold number of lives, he now felt he should have served his country in uniform. When this gray-haired advanced cancer patient told his wife about the plan, she quipped, "That's one heck of a midlife crisis. But, in fairness, I guess you can't afford a Maserati, and you don't have the nerve to take a mistress."

At first, the army wouldn't take him, but he pulled some strings with friends in high places. Amazingly, Trip endured army basic training as a fifty-four-year-old cancer patient who took fifty pills a day and had just completed chemotherapy. The army needed doctors, so he deployed to Iraq as medical liaison to commanding general George Casey. There he organized field medical programs and treated soldiers even while undergoing further rounds of chemo and coming under shelling during an insurgent ambush. He served two tours in Iraq and one in Afghanistan.

Promoted to colonel, Trip earned a reputation as an effective leader. Shortly after a scandal broke about inadequate care at Walter Reed Army Medical Center, President Bush named Trip the assistant secretary of Defense for Health Affairs. After he addressed the conditions at Walter Reed, the Defense Department awarded him its highest civilian honor, the Distinguished Public Service Medal. Returning to Houston, Trip founded a company that compiled health data for policy makers. He published papers on heart attacks, stroke, medical ethics, and nanotechnology. In 2009, he came out with a book-length tribute to medics killed in Iraq and Afghanistan. "Scoring" doesn't begin to account for what Trip accomplished.

It takes courage to be a patient and Trip Casscells was as courageous as anyone I've known. He had several cancer recurrences, and each time endured surgery or advanced chemotherapy. When his doctors ran out of treatments, he agreed to participate in a series of five clinical trials to buy time. This was a major contribution that helped pave the way for others.

No one would have criticized him if he'd simply retired. But that wasn't the Trip I knew. His example over the last eleven years of his life defies any attempt to "score" the costs of his treatment. Near the end, before he succumbed at age sixty, he was at peace: "God's given me time to kiss my family's tears away."

THE RIGHT WAY TO KEEP SCORE

I don't know what it cost to treat Trip Casscells's cancer or little Robin Bush's leukemia.* What I do know is that we've never accurately "scored" the value of treatments, the research behind them, and the lives they enable. They score zero according to the government system, which gives no credit to those lives' achievements or the people they motivated.

It's time we stopped thinking about research and treatment as just a cost. Let's also look at the social benefits side of the ledger. Consider the millions of cancer patients who were once expected to die

---

* You may remember my mentioning that President George W. Bush lost his three-year-old sister Robin to leukemia in the 1950s. Their father, George H. W. Bush, and their grandfather, Senator Prescott Bush, were men of substantial wealth and influence. But no amount of money could save Robin at a time when the parents of children diagnosed with leukemia were told to make the most of their short time together. The interval from playground to cemetery was as little as ninety days. Today, thanks to advanced therapies, these parents can be told to start saving for college. Put aside for a moment the priceless gift that survival is to a family. Consider only the cold economic fact that the child will grow up and contribute to the national economy in myriad ways through decades of employment and paying taxes. It's a good return on the investment in basic science that made lifesaving drugs for leukemia and many other diseases possible.

and who now live full, meaningful lives. They would fill every Major League Baseball stadium several times over. We all gain something when these lives are extended and enhanced. It's not just the added productivity in the economy, but also the human impact on family, friends, and caregivers.

The best investments we can make are in each other.

FIFTEEN

The New Wonder Drug: Prevention

During what I called my financial clinical trials period in the early 1970s, the Bendix Corporation ran a clever television commercial for their Fram oil filters. Hidden under the front end of a car in an auto repair shop, a mechanic explained he was replacing the car's main bearing. Then, as his grease-covered arm reached out to pick up a new Fram oil filter, he said, "If the guy who owns this car had paid four bucks for one of these, he wouldn't be paying me two hundred bucks for repairs."* Popping his head out from under the bumper, he delivered the punch line: "The choice is yours—you can pay me now . . . or pay me later."

---

* This is in 1972 dollars. Two hundred dollars then would be about $1,400 in 2023.

It's the same, of course, with your body. Take care of it now and your long-term healthcare costs will very likely be lower. Don't take care of it and you might not have a long term.

CRAZY STUFF

Cures and effective treatments for many diseases are wonderful. It's even better when we can prevent those diseases from occurring in the first place. As Amgen CEO Bob Bradway told me, "The next great drugs will be prediction and prevention." Looking at it that way, prevention is a wonder drug. The medical and scientific communities are increasingly recognizing that nutrition is an important component of that wonder drug.

It hasn't always been that way. This became clear at our 1994 CaP CURE Scientific Retreat in Santa Barbara. The program committee had created an agenda full of highly technical presentations about cancer. I personally invited Dr. David Heber, the respected director of the UCLA/NCI Clinical Nutrition Research Unit and editor in chief of the medical textbook *Nutritional Oncology*. That, it turned out, was an issue.

No one questioned David's qualifications as an experienced physician, professor of medicine, and author of many widely cited professional papers. It was the *subject* of his proposed lecture that bothered the program committee. "This conference is about hard science," said the committee chairman. "It's not about unproven theories of nutrition."

When I protested that there was evidence of links between nutrition and the prevention or progression of disease, he was dismissive. "Mike, we appreciate your help in supporting our research, but now you're telling us crazy stuff. If you think eating vegetables or anything else can prevent cancer, prove it." Eventually we reached a compromise. The committee agreed that Dr. Heber could speak briefly at lunch, but they would not list him on the official agenda. David gave a powerful talk about the effects of a low-fat diet on prostate cancer progression that changed many attendees' views about nutrition and cancer. The next year, he was part of the regular program.

At the time, anecdotal evidence *suggested* associations between diet and cancer; but no one could prove a clear causal effect. Technology didn't exist to study the cellular interactions between food and tumors. Today, thanks to advances in genomic sequencing and imaging, we can *prove* the link.

Even as far back as 1994, we'd seen studies showing wide variations in the incidence of certain diseases around the world. Hormone-driven cancers were relatively rare in countries like Japan where obesity was not widespread and consumption of red meat was low. Once such populations started to adopt a typical Western fast-food diet, the variations narrowed. When one of two Japanese brothers moved to the United States, the immigrant's children would usually develop a disease profile typical of people with European origins.

IT JUST AIN'T SO

The nexus between food and health is only the latest example of scientific proof lagging behind what we "know" from simple observation:

+ As early as the 1930s, some public health advocates were warning about the risks of smoking.* Yet cigarette sales kept rising for

---

* Concern about smoking actually goes back much further. In 1604, King James I of England described it as "a lothsome blacke stinking fume."

decades. During World War II, the US military distributed cigarettes to soldiers in ration kits on the theory that it would improve morale. Cigarette companies were among the largest print and broadcast advertisers. With evidence accumulating, the US surgeon general issued a 1964 report linking smoking and disease. Still, as late as 1986, the number-one brand in America was Marlboro.

+ In the 1970s, UCSF's Dr. Stanley Prusiner hypothesized that some cases of sudden onset dementia were caused by misfolded proteins that he called prions. The medical consensus ignored or dismissed his unproven and "dubious" theory of previously undescribed infections. Twenty years later, it earned him a Nobel Prize.

+ Until the 1980s, "everyone knew" that stomach ulcers were caused by a combination of emotional stress and a spicy diet. Two Australian scientists, Robin Warren and Barry Marshall, had a different idea—that a gastrointestinal pathogen caused ulcers. I remember an attendee at one of our medical meetings saying, "That's crazy. Who are these yobos and where did they go to school?"* In 2005, Warren and Marshall shared the Nobel Prize for their discovery of the real cause, a bacterium called *Helicobacter pylori.*

Early in life, I concluded that trying to change people's minds with logical arguments doesn't always work very well. The process of self-discovery is far more powerful. It's hard to shake people's biases by showing them evidence that they're wrong.

We're all subject to bias. As a child, I was sure that brussels sprouts weren't good for anything other than throwing at my little brother in food fights. Reading the scientific literature a half century later, I learned that Mom was right: This vegetable contains

---

* "Yobo" is Australian slang for an obnoxious, uncouth man.

sulforaphane, an antioxidant phytochemical with anticancer properties. (The concept of food as medicine is gaining traction. Some recent studies even suggest that specific foods, especially those that reduce inflammation, affect our moods and may slow the onset of dementia.)

The minds of doctors may be the hardest to change. As late as the 1970s, many of them continued to smoke. My advocacy of nutrition research in the 1990s was met with condescension if not outright derision. The medical profession's ideas about food as medicine finally began to evolve after reviewing the research we and others sponsored on the microbiome and the impact of diet on gene expression and mortality.

These examples of medical intransigence are nothing new. In the nineteenth century, doctors ridiculed the idea that washing their hands could help prevent lethal bacterial infections and that pre-operative skin antisepsis could make surgery safer. As Mark Twain said, "What gets us into trouble is not what we don't know. It's what we know for sure that just ain't so."

I don't mean to suggest that the eminent physicians and scientists participating in our early scientific retreats were closed-minded. They certainly weren't. But they demanded proof, not just theories. That's why we've tried hard to deliver proof by sponsoring rigorous scientific studies.

Work by Nicole Simone, MD, a PCF-supported professor at Thomas Jefferson University in Philadelphia, is transforming the standard of care for many cancer patients.* Dr. Simone's early work

---

* Dr. Simone's work builds in part on earlier studies by other PCF-supported investigators including Lorelei Mucci, ScD, MPH, a distinguished epidemiologist at Harvard Medical School and the Harvard T.H. Chan School of Public Health; and William Nelson, MD, PhD, a recognized leader in translational cancer research, director of the Johns Hopkins Sidney Kimmel Comprehensive Cancer Center and a professor in the Bloomberg

demonstrated that breast cancer patients who reduced calories by 25 percent experienced less toxicity from treatments, decreased tumor size, and fewer metastases. The lower caloric load altered their cell metabolism—especially in their guts—and made cancer cells more vulnerable to radiation and chemotherapy. Overall survival increased.*

More recent studies that use genomic and microbiome sequencing go beyond simple caloric restriction by marrying precision medicine with precision nutrition. This evolving scientific field is no longer limited to one-size-fits-all diets. It combines genetics, microbiome studies, eating times, exercise, food preparation, and more to create personalized anti-inflammatory diets matched to specific tumors in prostate, breast and endometrial cancers. As a result, an increasing number of primary care physicians are prescribing medically tailored meals.†

THE OBESITY CHALLENGE

Obesity is one of the greatest long-term public health challenges worldwide. It's not just the quantity of food, but also its quality. Americans eat less than half the recommended daily amount of fruits and vegetables while consuming *five times* the recommended limit of sugar. A 2014 study by Nobel laureate Elizabeth Blackburn,

---

School of Public Health at Johns Hopkins. Bill has long been a scientific advisor to the Prostate Cancer Foundation.

* See the monograph, "Fighting Cancer with Precision Nutrition," available at www .jefferson.edu.

† The PCF has published a "periodic table" of microbiome-friendly foods based on the familiar table of chemical elements you may have studied in high school. This periodic table of foods is reproduced at www.fastercuresbook.com.

a renowned cell biologist, showed that drinking two cans of sugary soda a day aged people's bodies by 4.6 years over a lifetime. When Dr. Blackburn joined me on a Milken Institute Global Conference panel the following year, she explained that a diet high in sugar has the effect of shortening our telomeres—the protective caps at the ends of chromosomes. Shorter telomeres indicate faster aging.

The effects of sugar can been seen dramatically in one of history's largest natural experiments—the dietary changes of more than a billion Chinese. Until a generation ago, diabetes was virtually unknown in China and was barely taught in Chinese medical schools. Now, a few decades after the invasion of fast foods, obesity and diabetes are endemic, especially in the major eastern cities. Today, more people in China have diabetes than in any other country.

Another natural experiment occurred in both of the twentieth century's world wars. During World War I, Americans were urged to "sacrifice" by eating more fruits and vegetables so that scarce sugar and fats could be sent to our troops. Meat, cheese, butter, cooking fats, and sugar were rationed in England during both wars. Meanwhile, naval blockades cut supplies of gasoline, forcing people to walk more. The result? Diabetes increased every year from 1905 to 1950 *except* for two periods: 1915–1918 and 1940–1945. During those war years, diabetes declined. Sad to say, most people don't get the connection.

GOOD BUGS

Obesity has multiple causes including lack of exercise, poor diet choices, hormone imbalances, emotional hunger, and defective signals from the brain. For many, however, the problem is in the gut. The trillions of microscopic colonists—mostly non-human bacteria, viruses, and fungi—in our digestive tract do far more than process food. This microbiome, which comprises the majority of our immune system, can help protect us from cancer, heart disease, and a long list of other conditions. When it gets out of balance, toxins can leak into your bloodstream, increase inflammation, and make you feel sick.*

We've sponsored many studies of the microbiome over the years and made more than a hundred presentations at conferences around the world. Interest in the field has grown enormously. What was a "crazy idea" at our first scientific retreat in 1994 has now become a cornerstone of academic discussions. At our latest retreat, about one-fifth of the panels related in some way to gut health.

The health effects of obesity are obvious. So is the economic impact. According to a 2019 Milken Institute study, the total cost to treat health conditions related to obesity, plus obesity's drag on job attendance and productivity, exceeds $1.4 trillion a year in the United States.† That's about twice what we spent on national defense. Other costs include the additional fuel airlines must purchase to carry heavier passengers and similar expenses in other industries.

Financial markets have reflected this effect. Several years ago, the Kraft Heinz Company and Nestlé were fairly comparable food

---

* Other than eating a healthy diet, clinicians warn against self-medicating in other ways by attempting to manipulate the microbiome, which can be a source of both beneficial and detrimental microbes. This is especially important during cancer therapy when certain gut microbes can stimulate the growth of cancer cells. Scientists are only beginning to understand the relationship between the microbiome and antibiotics although it appears that long-term use of these medicines could seriously damage your intestinal tract.

† That's just for obesity-related conditions. The total for twenty-four chronic diseases—nearly all preventable—is $3.7 trillion a year. The Milken Institute study estimated that 47 percent of chronic disease treatment costs relate to obesity. An obese person is 55 percent more likely to suffer from depression.

manufacturing companies. In 2017, Kraft's market capitalization was about $120 billion and Nestlé's was $230 billion. By November 2022, Kraft's market cap had *dropped* nearly two-thirds to $46 billion while Nestle's had *grown* to $296 billion. What happened? In 2017, Nestle hired a new CEO from the healthcare industry who announced that they would become a healthcare company. The initial public reaction was negative. One social media comment said, "First they make you sick with junk food; then they try to make money curing you." In short order, Nestle acquired a plant-based food company, a vitamin maker, a plant-based snack food business, and a biopharmaceutical company. They cut the salt and sugar in many other products and sold their ice cream and candy businesses. The market got the message and adjusted corporate values to where the future lies.

Since those transactions in 2017, the ratio of Nestle's equity value compared to Kraft's has grown from about 2:1 to more than 6:1. It's not that Kraft didn't have sophisticated owners—their controlling stockholders are G3 Capital of Brazil and the legendary investor Warren Buffett. But their knowledge of markets didn't help the company because they didn't adequately adjust to the new knowledge of health.

OUR SELF-DISCOVERY STRATEGY

The private dining room in the United States Senate and a schoolroom in Anacostia, one of Washington, DC's poorest neighborhoods, are a few miles from each other and a world apart on the spectrum of exclusivity. Yet each was a forum for letting self-discovery achieve what no lecture from me could have done.

During a cooking demonstration at an Anacostia school, several kids were happy to join me to make chocolate pudding. They were less sure when I shook a jiggling container of high-protein silken tofu into a bowl. One of the youngsters said it looked like a quivering blob from outer space. None of them would get near the stuff until we gave them gloves. But after they mixed the ingredients and tasted the pudding, one of them asked if he could lick the pan. We had similar results with a group of kids at Lake Tahoe in a cooking demonstration that was covered by CNN.

Over the week before our 1998 March on Washington, we received permission to replace many items on the menu of the Senate dining room. Ted Stevens and a few other senators helped us arrange this switch, but most senators didn't know about it. (A few choices remained sacrosanct—the dining staff wouldn't let us change the Boston cream pie or mess with an item that had been on the menu since the founding of the republic: US Senate Navy Bean Soup.) Later, when we announced what we'd done, there was bipartisan agreement that our healthier versions of traditional dishes were as good as the "real thing."

We had similar excellent results at other locations including Dole Foods headquarters, where we replaced several cafeteria items for a week. On another occasion, when I was interviewed by ABC television host Barbara Walters on the *20/20* program, we switched a number of ingredients on the menu at the network's commissary in New York. Only a few diners made comments. One said that our thin-crust pizza was great—they finally got it right. He didn't know it was vegetarian. There was some confusion about the tofu hot dogs—people didn't like them because they had been boiled by the cafeteria instead of grilling as we specified.

For a few hours one afternoon, a Philly cheesesteak vendor allowed us to substitute a meatless version of my old favorite at his downtown Philadelphia stand. It was made with seitan (a meat analogue derived from wheat gluten), onions, vegan cheese, mushrooms, peppers, and spices on a roll. Most customers didn't even notice the changed ingredients. A few said, "It tastes good. Different, but good."

These were small victories, but they're symbolic of what we can do with greater focus on that wonder drug called prevention.

SIXTEEN

What Are the Alternatives?

A few months after my cancer diagnosis, Rosey Grier asked if I'd be willing to speak at his church in South Los Angeles. The Crenshaw Christian Center was at the time the largest domed sanctuary in the United States. Multiple services were needed to accommodate almost thirty thousand primarily African American congregants. Thousands more watched broadcasts of Sunday services on television.

That Sunday, Rosey introduced me to the pastor, the charismatic Reverend Frederick K. C. Price, and took me to several classrooms on the Crenshaw campus, where I spoke to groups of kids about health and prevention. Then I delivered what seemed to me like a rousing talk from the pulpit, thanked everyone, and prepared to leave. That's when the pastor said, "Brother Michael, please accept the laying on of hands to help you heal from your illness."

I assumed he would do something like put his hand on my

shoulder and say a blessing for me. Nothing had prepared me for what came next. Reverend Price beckoned me to stand in the center aisle where about a dozen men gathered around me in a circle. Each in turn came forward to touch me as they all prayed that I would receive the Spirit of the Lord. The entire congregation joined in with joyous hymns and prayers for my recovery. Shouts of "Praise the Lord" echoed off the walls of the cavernous structure. My friend Deepak Chopra once told me there's a healing force in the world that a group of people can focus onto one person. But this was an experience unlike anything I'd ever imagined. The place was rocking! It was incredibly emotional, and I'm sure it helped energize my immune system.

That Sunday began with my thinking I'd share some knowledge with this group as a favor to Rosey. Instead, I became the student and was humbly grateful.

NO FALSE HOPES

These intercessions on my behalf occurred when we were all working hard to build CaP CURE as a new type of medical research organization. It was crucial work, yet I also needed to focus on my own health because I couldn't help others in the future without a future of my own. My terminal prognosis called for lifestyle changes.

Let me say upfront that I am a firm believer in traditional Western medicine. I owe my life to it. When a patient starts talking about alternative or complementary therapies, many medical professionals roll their eyes.* They know the danger in offering false hopes. Today's

---

* An NCI official once told me the two groups they most despise are tobacco companies and hucksters who peddle worthless nostrums to cancer patients.

internet contains far too much misleading and outright dangerous information. In the middle stands the practice of *responsible* alternative medicine based on rigorous science that emphasizes prevention. The National Center for Complementary and Integrative Health within the NIH helps separate promising approaches from quackery.

In 1993, I determined to explore every alternative option that was generally considered safe. Dozens of my friends and relatives had passively followed the traditional regimens of Western medicine . . . and every one of them had died. What else could I do that they had not? I'd already sworn off high-fat foods and stuck to my drab diet. A single serving of "light" peanut butter exceeded my daily fat allowance of nine grams. While I felt virtuous eating a salad of mixed greens, even a small amount of the usual dressings put me over the limit.

I started studying Eastern medicine and its concept of energizing the human body. Clearly, my health had suffered from all those years eating fatty and sugar-laden foods, all the meals consumed in haste. I began by exploring and, in some cases, embracing several alternative concepts: meditation, sesame oil massages, aromatherapy, and yoga. These nontraditional methods seemed at worst harmless and might help.

Studies supported by CaP CURE showed that sunlight and the vitamin D it produces help reduce the growth of prostate cancer. The studies also found a higher incidence of hormone-related cancers in northern Europe and the northern United States than in sunnier southern areas. I thought back to all those long days in my windowless New York office, all those winter mornings setting off for work in darkness and returning in darkness. I had seen no more daylight than a hibernating bear. Even when I moved back to sunny LA, for much of the year, I left for work before dawn and returned after sunset. It was time to take more daytime walks.

GOTHIC REVIVAL

In April 1993, at the suggestion of Deepak Chopra, Lori and I joined him for a week at the Maharishi Ayurveda Center in Lancaster, Massachusetts. While Lori drove the one-hour trip from the airport, I closed my eyes and meditated, visualizing my T cells as little Pac-Men gobbling up cancer cells.

It was 10:00 p.m., raining and foggy by the time our car approached the center and we turned into a long entrance drive. "I can hardly see," said Lori as the wipers stuttered across the windshield. When the car lurched to a stop, my eyes popped open, and in the headlights, I could pick out the shadows of drenched bushes and low-hanging branches. Lori turned to me apprehensively and described the ornate Gothic building looming over us as something out of Edgar Allan Poe's *The Fall of the House of Usher*. It looked haunted.

After everything we'd been through with my diagnosis, trips to medical centers, and cancer treatments, we'd been looking forward to several days of stress-reducing programs. Our initial impression was hardly stress-free. An attendant led us up a creaking staircase to an overheated second-floor room filled with a strong aroma of incense. Lori tried in vain to open the locked window. I thought the incense smelled wonderful, but Lori said it was giving her a headache. An Amrit paste and pill by our bedside were to help with sleep. I ate my paste and tossed down the pill. Lori chose not to take hers.

The next morning, we were introduced to the nutritional program, which was strictly vegetarian. To drink, there was a choice of tepid apple juice, warm water, or hot herbal tea. All sources of caffeine were forbidden. Cold drinks, cold food, and caffeine were considered bad for the digestive system. Then, an Ayurveda physician examined us to determine our "dosha," or character type, believed to be responsible for physical and mental health. This would guide the treatment regimens. The three doshas—Vata, Kapha, and Pitta—go from thin, Type-A personalities along a spectrum to the obese and lethargic. Most people are a combination. Mine came out Vata/Pitta.

The week's lectures and exercise programs were built on the consciousness-based teachings of Vedic science. Much of it made sense to me as an alternative approach. Later, we brought a young physician trained in both Western and Ayurveda medicine into our house for several months. Early in the morning and late at night, we worked on breathing techniques, herbal therapy, meditation, and yoga.

This began my adoption of a wide range of non-Western medicine. I went to Russia on a family trip in the summer of 1994 and met with a healer; then a business trip to China where I interacted with qi doctors.* It seemed important to connect the mind with the body. I had a fountain installed outside the windows of my library so that reading would be accompanied by the soothing sounds of flowing water.

There was even time to smell the flowers, literally, as Lori and I took a vacation that included a visit to the beautiful Keukenhof Gardens in Holland. Did all this help? Maybe. I was willing to try anything that had potential. To this day, I take my prescribed medications, eat a very healthy diet, exercise, and try to keep everything in

---

* Some years later during a family adventure vacation in northern Brazil, I channeled Sean Connery in the movie *Medicine Man*. The plot involved a search for some substance in the jungle that gave the native population immunity to various diseases. Our guide pointed out one plant he said protects against malaria. Perhaps it does—he seemed perfectly healthy despite wearing no shirt as we trudged through swarms of mosquitos. Or perhaps, I speculated, the rich Amazonian ecosystem might even contain some other substance to energize the immune system and prevent cancer. We must have looked like a Monty Python comedy troupe—the guide in nothing but shorts; Lori in an all-white outfit; and I dressed totally in black from my wide-brimmed hat to dark hiking shoes. If nearby critters wanted to feast on someone for lunch, I hoped my achromatic garb would discourage them.

perspective. Another habit that emerged from this period: speaking to other patients every day. It's as rewarding for me as it is for them.*

THE TASTE FOR LIVING

So far, so good. But every unappealing bowl of plain raw vegetables tempted me to slip back to the old ways. There was no joy in eating anymore. My mind would wander: *I sure could go for a Top Dog frankfurter or a big chef's salad with slices of meat and lots of creamy Thousand Island dressing!*

This reminded me of some business interactions a decade earlier when East Coast clients would visit to meet with me in our California offices. We were not far from the Pritikin Longevity Center, which offered two-and four-week programs of strenuous exercise and stringent low-fat, low-calorie diets designed to reduce weight, reverse heart disease, and extend life. Some of our customers combined a West Coast business trip with a course at Pritikin.

The original Pritikin diet (which has since been improved) tried to approximate the eating patterns of primitive peoples by severely restricting calories and eliminating most fats, sugar, dairy, salt, alcohol, and caffeine. This clearly had health benefits, but it took monumental self-discipline to follow the strict Pritikin rules. Our clients soon grew tired of healthy-but-unappetizing food and would sometimes sneak out to enjoy our tasty-but-unhealthy alternatives.

After two years of deprivation, I understood how those clients felt when they guiltily scarfed down cheeseburgers or glazed doughnuts and coffee. But with my cancer apparently in remission, I was deter-

* The best time to talk to patients is soon after they've received a diagnosis or reoccurrence. That's when they're most receptive to objective advice.

mined to maintain my resolve if only I could find a diet that was both healthy and satisfying. I consulted a number of scientists who had studied the link between diet and cancer; then began a worldwide search for someone who would incorporate our nutritional research into recipes that could actually be enjoyed. The search led to Beth Ginsberg, an accomplished chef who specialized in healthy cuisine. Her cooking wasn't anything like what I had grudgingly come to accept as part of my recovery. She could make delicious versions of my old favorites by substituting different ingredients to make them healthy.

Like many others, I'd tried a variety of "health foods" including some gray slabs of fake "meat" that looked and tasted like cardboard. Eating was more a burden than a pleasure. I gave Beth an assignment: Try to produce my favorite foods with 90 to 95 percent of the fat and calories removed—things like Philadelphia cheesesteak, Caesar salad, chili, Reubens, and chocolate pudding. The foods must taste, smell, and look like the original versions.

As Beth experimented with new recipes, I served as official food tester. Not everything could be adapted successfully, as we learned from her attempt to make a healthy version of caramel corn. It tasted good, but my teeth stuck together so firmly I almost pulled some molars out of their sockets trying to pry them apart!

There were also great successes. Beth turned my medicinal soy protein shakes into delicious fruit smoothies that reminded me of the Swiss Orange Chip ice cream I used to order at Swensen's in Berkeley. It was loaded with soy protein and other potential cancer fighters like lemon and orange zest.

Good nutrition—good *tasty* nutrition—was an important part of my recovery. Another part was the mind-body connection. Like Marcel Proust, for whom the aroma of fresh madeleine cakes triggered joyous memories of childhood, I found a similar trigger in the smells of pine needles and the salty air of the seashore. Some of the happiest days of my younger years began with early morning walks when Dad and I hiked among the trees at Lake Arrowhead. The smell of pine needles always thrusts me back to those boyhood days. Later tests showed that this aromatherapy actually raised my cancer-fighting T-cell count.

During my early recovery from cancer, I built a house on the north shore of Lake Tahoe and surrounded it with pine and incense cedar trees, flowers, and walking paths to reproduce childhood memories. My rebirth was personal, but the lifestyle concepts could be shared widely. In 1996, I celebrated my fiftieth birthday by inviting about two hundred longtime friends, health leaders, philanthropists, and CEOs to join me in Tahoe. Over three days, we focused on nutrition, wellness, and other healthy topics while enjoying the mountain air, great food, and some entertaining quizzes. On the program were four well-known physician-authors who had never previously been together: Andrew Weil, Dean Ornish, Deepak Chopra, and David Heber.

Dr. Weil spoke about the benefits of a plant-based diet; Dr. Ornish explained that certain lifestyle changes, including relaxation and loving touches, can help reverse chronic diseases; Dr. Chopra said meditation can mobilize the immune system; and Dr. Heber went into detail on the ways soy and other sources of isoflavones improve the microbiome's environment to reduce cancer risk. Their talks reinforced my views of Ayurvedic medicine, diet, meditation, massages, aromatherapy, and other nontraditional approaches as supplements to my ongoing standard treatments.*

---

* A few years ago, Lori and I participated in a lifestyle change program created by Dean Ornish at UCLA. We also underwent exhaustive testing at what was then called the J. Craig Venter Institute in La Jolla, California, to determine if we had genetic predispositions to cancer that might be inherited by succeeding generations. (The Institute later became part of UC San Diego.) They sequenced our DNA and ran dozens of sophisticated

Rather than lecture the guests or tell them the food was good for them because of its different ingredients, we let Beth's delicious meals deliver the message.*

COOKBOOKS

In 1998, after more than three years of testing and research, CaP CURE published *The Taste for Living Cookbook: Mike Milken's Favorite Recipes for Fighting Cancer*, combining nutritional guidelines with tasty, thoroughly tested, easy-to-prepare recipes. In this first of two cookbooks, Beth worked with nutritionists and medical research scientists to develop healthier versions of such traditionally high-fat foods as puddings, cakes, sauce-laden pastas, cheese-based dishes, and much more.

The cookbook also included such practical information as how to make sense of a food label. It stressed the point that it isn't just the bad stuff in our diets that puts us at risk—it's also what we don't eat that contributes to disease. An afterword by Dr. Donald Coffey from Johns Hopkins Hospital explained how different foods can either

---

tests of blood, urine, stool, and microbiomes. We were pleased to learn that the results showed nothing relevant in our genes. In particular, I had no apparent predisposition to prostate cancer. I concluded that excessive aggravation and stress in prior decades may have weakened my immune system and made me more vulnerable to cancer.

* In most cases where we substituted healthier ingredients, people didn't know the difference. I set out to prove this one day when I'd had enough of Lew Solmon teasing me about what he called my "rabbit food" lunches. Dr. Lewis Solmon was the first president of the Milken Institute and he loved Reuben sandwiches—the more fatty corned beef, Swiss cheese, and Russian dressing the better. Beth Ginsberg and I hatched a plan to substitute healthier ingredients in his Reuben without telling him. Later, when Beth asked if he enjoyed the sandwich, he said it was very good—just the way he likes it. He couldn't believe it when she explained that it contained a tempeh meat analogue, fat-free soy cheese, and Thousand Island dressing made with silken tofu.

damage our health or protect us. A year later, we published *The Taste for Living World Cookbook* with favorite recipes for fighting heart disease and cancer gathered from our travels around the world. (We did omit one dish Lori and I encountered near the Great Wall of China—grilled scorpion!)*

The Taste for Living cookbook became a bestseller, buoyed by a cover feature in *Business Week* and by several national television appearances. The day after Barbara Walters featured my story on ABC's 20/20, the cookbook was the fourth-best-selling book on Amazon. I also discussed nutrition on *The Charlie Rose Show* and *Access Hollywood*, among others, and appeared with Cindy Crawford on *Larry King Live* to discuss healthy eating. The resulting publicity not only helped sell cookbooks; it also encouraged people to think about what they ate and to get involved in debates about such food-related matters as school lunches, hospital trays, and airline meals.

The cookbooks and CaP CURE's research supported each other. Recipes were based on the results of CaP CURE–supported clinical trials. Proceeds from the cookbooks were being returned to support additional research. Readers could find cancer-fighting meals created with low-fat or soy-based ingredients—spaghetti Bolognese, quiche Lorraine, and egg rolls—that didn't taste like they were created in a laboratory. And they could learn not only cooking techniques, but *why* certain ingredients were good for them.

---

* Our studies of foods around the world supported one theory of why African Americans have relatively high incidences of colon, prostate, and breast cancer. East Africans traditionally ate a diet that included meat, butter, and milk—all high in fat and low in fiber. But most African Americans trace their origins to *West* Africa, where the diet in the pre-slavery era consisted mostly of high-fiber, plant-based foods such as root vegetables, grains, fruits, and greens. After eons of evolution on the African continent, a few hundred years in North America is too short a time for their genes to adapt to a fat-laden American diet replete with refined sugars and fried foods.

My three-pronged approach—traditional medicine, nutritional therapies, and Ayurvedic techniques—seemed to be effective. Now it was time to broaden the focus.

HEALTHY PEOPLE, HEALTHY PLANET

At the 2005 Milken Institute Global Conference, Al Gore paced nervously backstage just before being introduced to a packed ballroom. "Are you confident," asked the former vice president, "they can handle all my slides, videos, and audio effects?" We assured him that the technical crew was first-rate. Still, with more than three hundred slides interspersed with dramatic video and booming sound, all projected in a forty-five-minute presentation on multiple screens, there was no room for error.

It went perfectly and the audience was impressed with Al's argument that climate change is real, man-made, and potentially cataclysmic. Seated in the audience was documentary filmmaker Davis Guggenheim, who later turned the presentation into *An Inconvenient Truth*, the Academy Award–winning documentary that had a powerful impact on the climate change debate.

Several years later, James Cameron, the Oscar-winning director of *Avatar*, *Titanic*, and other Hollywood blockbusters, stood on the same stage at the Global Conference with his wife, environmental advocate Suzy Amis Cameron. The Camerons presented a compelling case for plant-based diets, not only because they're healthier, but also because they can help save the planet. According to studies cited by the Camerons, children raised on a plant-based diet grow taller and have higher IQs. They called the idea that we must eat meat to get adequate protein "a complete myth." Yet they recognized the difficulty of convincing people to change. So they proposed a gradual process:

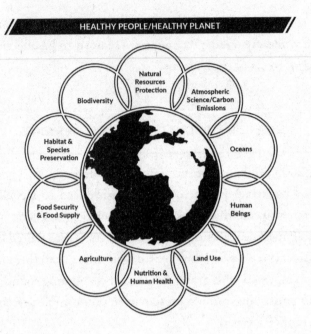

HEALTHY PEOPLE/HEALTHY PLANET

Go ahead and eat your bacon cheeseburger if you must; but have one meal a day that's entirely plant-based. Aside from your own health benefits, you'll save more than 194,000 gallons of water a year and the carbon equivalent of driving three thousand miles.

Fast-forward a few more years and the Sheth Sangreal Foundation joined the Milken Institute to convene an important retreat for philanthropic leaders in the conservation movement. Sangreal's cofounder, Brian Sheth, and I led a wide range of discussions about solutions to the crisis in biodiversity.

Each of these Milken Institute programs carried forward a theme we've emphasized since the mid-1990s when CaP CURE first highlighted the links between what we eat and our environment. We've long stressed the point that environmental health and human health must be considered part of the same issue.

More recently, the Institute and the Motsepe Foundation announced the Milken-Motsepe Prize in AgriTech. This initiative addresses the fact that the world population is expected to reach 8.5 billion by 2030 with most of the growth in sub-Saharan Africa. Food availability in that region will have to grow by 50 percent, yet agricultural productivity growth in most African nations is far below that of other developing countries. Agricultural technology (AgriTech) can greatly increase crop yields, farm productivity, plant and animal health, sustainability, and waste reduction. The Milken-Motsepe Prize is a $2 million global competition for solutions to problems faced by farmers on small to medium-sized African farms. It provides incentives for global innovators to develop Fourth Industrial Revolution (4IR) technologies—artificial intelligence, 3D printing, robotics, and more—that will accelerate progress on the first two sustainable development goals of the United Nations: no poverty and zero hunger.

In the initial competition round, more than 3,300 applicants from 105 countries across six continents registered to submit ideas that can help farmers, alleviate poverty, and transform food systems. Twenty-five finalists were chosen in early 2022. Each finalist team received $10,000 to develop and test their designs. The grand prize winner will receive $1 million with additional prize money to second and third place winners.

INNOVATIVE SOLUTIONS

This little blue planet we live on is all we have. Someday far in the future, humans may inhabit other planets. For now there's nowhere else to go, so we'd better take care of what we have. Much as we would like to eliminate use of fossil fuels, there is no practical way to do so in the foreseeable future. Until then, progress on cleaner sources of energy will require an "all-of-the-above" approach incorporating wind, solar, biomass, nuclear, geothermal, heating-cooling-storage efficiencies, greener fuels like hydrogen and ammonia, hydropower, improved food production, and some technology breakthroughs still to be developed. Entrepreneurial ingenuity offers endless possibilities for taking care of our planet.

Several years ago, I saw many intriguing examples of that ingenuity on a daylong visit to a natural products expo in Anaheim, California. Among the three thousand exhibitors was a company called Apeel Sciences that uses material from the seeds, peels, and pulp of fruits and vegetables to seal moisture in and keep oxygen out. This invisible layer is tasteless and odorless. It keeps food fresh twice as long through the supply chain. This means growers can pick the food closer to its maximum nutrition level. And it eliminates the plastic pollution of regular food wraps.

Other exhibitors at the food expo showed "tuna" and other types of seafood analogues from specially grown tomatoes. Another start-up claims to have perfected 3D-printed "salmon" fillets with the same taste, color, and consistency as fish while using only plant materials. These products are made without antibiotics and could someday help restore nature's balance in overfished oceans. During my tour in Anaheim, I invited several companies to present their concepts at Milken Institute conferences around the world.

The scope of today's industrial agriculture is huge: seventy-two billion farm animals plus well over a hundred billion fish are killed each year to feed us. We pump many of them full of antibiotics—twice as much as used on humans—to keep them from getting sick. A third of the world's land area is devoted to agriculture. That produces nearly a third of the heat-trapping gases that are warming the planet.

A partial solution is vertical farming, an intriguing land-preservation practice that we've featured at our conferences in the United States, the Middle East, and Singapore. Fruits and vegetables can now be grown in urban areas—projects that provide healthy food and good jobs close to home. Among the many advantages of vertical farming:

+ Crops are planted in tall buildings under LED lights that are 75 to 95 percent more efficient than incandescent lights.

+ These crops use a tiny fraction of the water required for traditional farming.

+ Since there are no soil contaminants, pesticides are unnecessary.

+ Vertical farmers using computers to control every indoor environmental variable are able to measure the nutritional content of their plants far more effectively.

+ Because crops are planted vertically, far less land is needed.

+ Crops can be planted and rotated all year without regard to weather.

+ Bacterial contamination from nearby animal farms and industries is eliminated.

+ Transportation costs and its pollution are reduced because food is produced closer to where it's consumed.

Vertical farms are far more efficient than horizontal greenhouse operations that can spread over hundreds of acres. Their major downside is the energy, often from fossil fuels, that provide heat and electricity. Advanced designs, including exterior solar panels and placement near sources of industrial waste heat, will mitigate that problem. Meanwhile, they offer consumers safe, more nutritious food with a fraction of the environmental impact of food from animals.

Plant-based versions of meat, fish, eggs, and dairy products provide one of the closest links between healthy people and a healthy planet. That's not to say that all vegetarian foods are "healthy"—many contain high amounts of saturated fats and sodium. But two main types of substitute-protein foods are showing much progress.

Beef analogues are made from such ingredients as pea protein, vegetable oils, mushrooms, potato starch, and beet juice that replace the muscle and fat from animals. It's better for the environment, and after many disappointing early attempts to replicate the taste and "mouthfeel" of meat, the products have started to approach the appeal of the real thing.

The other substitute is real meat, at least in terms of DNA. Instead of raising—and then killing—a cow, pig, chicken, or fish with all the attendant environmental destruction, scientists grow the product in a lab from animal cells. Nutritionally, this "cultured" meat is indistinguishable from the flesh of a slaughtered animal, but no animals are harmed and no methane released in its production. The required water, land, fertilizer, pesticides, and energy is minimal or eliminated. Considering that it takes at least 1,800 gallons of water to produce one pound of meat from a farm, the environmental benefits are substantial. According to the highly regarded book *Drawdown*, improved land use is one of the best ways to reduce air pollution.[*]

For now, the major barrier to meat replacements is cost, although that's declining rapidly. There are also regulatory hurdles that manufacturers will eventually overcome. These things are scaling up fast, which is causing the chain of animal production to evolve. Since

---

[*] Paul Hawken, ed. *Drawdown: The Most Comprehensive Plan Ever Proposed to Reverse Global Warming*, (Penguin, 2017). My friend Craig McCaw, whose cell-phone business I helped finance in the 1980s, later joined the board of the Nature Conservancy and supported many conservation programs advocated in *Drawdown*. The book notes a long list of technologies that can slow or reverse environmental destruction. Half of these technologies relate to food including refrigeration, food waste reduction, diet changes, forest preservation, and land-use efficiency.

Americans eat five times as much meat as in 1940, the impact can be substantial.*

Switching to a plant-based diet doesn't mean we have to deprive ourselves. A growing number of restaurants, at every price level, offer delicious meatless meals.

MEETING THE ENVIRONMENTAL CHALLENGE

Technology that addresses environmental challenges is moving quickly. We need more advanced technologies and more public support to save the planet. Wetlands, forests, grasslands—and the species that inhabit them—are disappearing. Meanwhile, the earth's population will continue to increase, at least for several decades, with much of the increase in Africa. Within a century, Nigeria is projected to have a larger population than China. The challenges of providing more people with meaningful jobs, nutritious food, clean water and good healthcare will be daunting. To do so, we must simultaneously protect the planet and create economic growth.

I'm optimistic that we can do it.

---

* Robert Paarlberg, "The Environmental Upside of Modern Farming," *Wall Street Journal*, February 5, 2021.

SEVENTEEN

FasterCures

In 2003, the food in the National Cancer Institute cafeteria was no more appetizing or healthy than it had been thirty years earlier when I began visiting NCI directors. That fact may not be central to the NCI's mission, but ten years after CaP CURE's first nutrition studies, it seemed symbolic of the government's slow-moving bureaucracy. There was hope, however, because President Bush had recently named my friend and colleague, Andy von Eschenbach, to head the agency.*

From his expansive Bethesda office, the director wielded broad authority, managing some four thousand employees and overseeing billions of dollars in cancer research funding. What thwarted his plans, Andy told me, was the inaccessibility of data: "The Kellogg

---

* Previously, I'd had productive relationships with former NCI directors Vincent DeVita, Samuel Broder, and Richard Klausner, all of whom had participated in our 1995 Cancer Summit. The relationship with Andy was closer, however, because of our shared experiences and his role on my clinical treatment team.

Company can track more information about a box of cereal than I can about a cancer patient."

I understood his frustration—access to good data had always been a central component of my work. Success in high school debate tournaments, in college studies of credit history, in attacking Wall Street's back-office problems, and in guiding CaP CURE's research initiatives starting in 1993—all depended on the right data.

Andy was well aware of what we'd achieved and now he was asking me for ideas about how similar concepts could be applied in his agency. I told him we were about to expand the mission of the organization that had been called CaP CURE for ten years and we'd be increasing our focus on data collection and many other barriers to medical research progress. Our understanding of the links among diseases had evolved over a decade—the lines between different cancers was blurring as investigators increasingly began to look at genomic similarities across diseases.

COAST TO COAST

A major expansion of our healthcare efforts required headquarters operations on both coasts. With offices in Washington, DC, we could more effectively contribute to the national discussion of health issues than one operating only from our Santa Monica base. We renamed the part of CaP CURE focused on prostate cancer as the Prostate Cancer Foundation (PCF), and assigned people working on all diseases to a new organization initially called the Center for Accelerating Medical Solutions. Then, at the suggestion of my co-author, Geoffrey Moore, we changed it to *FasterCures*.[*]

---

[*] A third organization—an outside group called C-Change—was founded in 1998 "to eliminate cancer as a major public health problem by leveraging the expertise and resources

Expanding CaP CURE wasn't just a matter of revising the organization chart, leasing new offices, and hiring more people. Many dedicated CaP CURE professionals were heavily invested in their expanding mission. After eleven years, it can be emotionally difficult to hand off part of that mission to a new group. But there was more than enough work for everyone, and we were able to manage the transition with minimal disruption.

Of approximately ten thousand diseases that have been identified worldwide, only five hundred have effective treatments. A new treatment can cost more than $1 billion to develop. It was obvious we needed to pick up the pace of development, lower the cost, and get therapies to patients as fast as possible. In other words, *time equals lives*. Washington didn't need another think tank. What it needed— or more accurately, what patients needed—was an *action tank*.

The more success the PCF had in developing improved therapies for prostate cancer, the more it began to contribute to solutions for other cancers and even for other noncancerous diseases. (Some of its important early research discoveries contributed to therapies for COVID-19.) Ever since the establishment of CaP CURE in 1993, we had shared our work with other disease groups such as the Multiple Myeloma Research Foundation (MMRF).* Most diseases, however,

---

of a unique multi-sector membership." For a while, we thought this group, originally called the National Dialogue on Cancer, would take some responsibility for the broad campaign against all cancers. However, a few years later, after attending a C-Change meeting, I concluded they weren't going to have a major impact on new treatments. They acted like the United Nations and just weren't focused on the right goals. As Dr. David Feinberg, my fellow *FasterCures* advisory board member and CEO of Cerner Corporation, the electronic health records company, puts it, "Some people want to shorten the line at Blockbuster Video; others want to invent Netflix." C-Change stopped operations at the end of 2016.

* The MMRF was founded 1998 by Kathy Giusti, a senior business executive, and her twin sister, Karen Andrews. Kathy is a cancer survivor, a member of the Harvard Business School faculty, and a highly effective leader of global efforts to accelerate precision med-

lacked this kind of effective research and advocacy organization. We addressed that issue by creating the TRAIN program—The Research Acceleration and Innovation Network—in 2005.*

The acronym is more than coincidental. Our first leader at *Faster-Cures* was Greg Simon, a visionary strategist who had been chief domestic policy advisor to Vice President Al Gore. Greg often used the analogy of a train. Modern railroad technology has produced trains that reach speeds greater than 250 miles per hour; yet in the United States, the average train chugs along at 55 miles per hour—exactly the same average speed as a century ago. Why? It's the tracks. The engines may be more powerful and the cars more streamlined, but without upgraded tracks, speed can't increase. It's the same with medical science: We've produced dazzling twenty-first-century advances, but the "tracks" between the laboratory bench and the patient bedside were conceived in the nineteenth century.

TRAIN is an affinity network of disease-specific foundations interested in taking a more strategic and entrepreneurial approach—sometimes called venture philanthropy—to upgrading the scientific tracks. We regularly bring together dozens of forward-thinking foundations so they can learn from each other, find relevant resources, and share their novel solutions with the rest of the medical research system. These organizations have rejected the old "spray-and-pray" method of funding medical science. As disruptive philanthropists who insist on results and accountability, they're actively involved at every stage.

---

icine. Her work through the MMRF helped sequence the myeloma gene and define the molecular subtypes of the disease. The MMRF has long been an active participant in our *FasterCures* research network.

* After media executive Sumner Redstone made a generous grant to expand the TRAIN program, we began calling it The *Redstone* Acceleration and Innovation Network. He was one of a number of philanthropists whose businesses I had financed years earlier who now made transformative gifts to advance our medical research programs.

FasterCures created new ways to link biomedical groups. Nearly every month, we convened meetings on such subjects as the status of medical informatics, innovation in disease research, case studies of progress against AIDS, and the transformation of clinical medicine from reactive to predictive. Each year, the Milken Institute Global Conference included dozens of panels on health-related topics including an annual session I moderated with several Nobel laureates in medicine.

In addition to convening long-established organizations, *Faster-Cures* reached out to founders of several recently established or planned groups to discuss our unique model. These included Michael J. Fox who, with Deborah Brooks, launched his eponymous Parkinson's Research Foundation (2000); Neal Kassell of the Focused Ultrasound Foundation (2006); and others. I gave speeches at meetings of several groups including those working on lung cancer, childhood diabetes and breast cancer. It's worthwhile, I said, to offer information and comfort to worried patients; but it's equally important to strengthen the research infrastructure.

FasterCures has helped to:
  » Improve public-private collaboration.
  » Speed adoption of new technologies.
  » Give patients a greater voice.
  » Increase federal science budgets.
  » Encourage biomedical careers.
  » Improve clinical trials participation.
  » Accelerate translational research.
  » Reduce grant-making bureaucracy.
  » Speed new drug approvals.
  » Update physician training.
  » Enhance medical-outcomes data.
  » Spotlight antimicrobial resistance.
  » Promote international research.

MRA

One morning early in 2007, I received a call from a longtime friend Debra Black, whose husband, Leon, had worked with me on financing companies beginning in the 1970s. Debra, a Tony Award–winning Broadway producer, got right to the point: "Mike, I've been diagnosed with melanoma and the cancer is fairly advanced. I know you've been involved in melanoma research, so you're the first person I thought of turning to for advice." As we spoke, I sensed in Debra the concerns of a patient and the determination of a committed philanthropist. I quickly connected her with various resources including Dr. Don Morton, who had treated my father and whose research we continued to support.

Debra and Leon were well aware of the Prostate Cancer Foundation's transformative impact on that disease and wanted to expand the field of melanoma studies based on the PCF model. I suggested that before they did anything, we should ask a *FasterCures* group called the Philanthropy Advisory Service (PAS) to conduct a rapid-but-thorough study of everything going on in melanoma worldwide.

With the results of the PAS study in hand, the Blacks said they would commit substantial funds to get a new organization started. The result was the Melanoma Research Alliance (MRA), which was initially organized under the auspices of the Milken Institute. With help from Milken Institute, PCF, and *FasterCures* executives who agreed to serve on the MRA board, this new disease-specific research organization had a big head start. Today, the MRA is one of more than a hundred TRAIN members and has become the world's largest private funder of research on deadly skin cancers. The studies it has supported with more than $150 million in grants stand behind fifteen new FDA-approved treatments that have saved thousands of lives.*

PATIENTS AT THE CENTER

From the earliest days of the TRAIN program, Greg Simon urged its member organizations not to waste resources competing with each other for donors, NIH grants, and publicity. They should focus on changing the biology of their specific diseases while *FasterCures* worked to enlarge the overall resource pie so everyone would receive a larger slice. Most importantly, we would focus on changing a culture in medical science that inhibited innovation. Specifically, we called for greater data sharing among research groups, increased use of electronic medical records, support for young researchers, a willingness to take more risks, and expanded budgets for government science agencies.

We had interacted with President Clinton since 1993, when he spoke to a CaP CURE meeting by telephone, and we maintained a close relationship with the White House through our efforts to pass the 1997 FDA Modernization Act and the doubling of the NIH budget beginning in 1998. Greg Simon had been working with Vice President Gore in the White House for much of that period. Now he led *FasterCures*, which built on everything we'd learned at CaP CURE, the lessons and momentum of the 1998

---

* In 2019, I attended an event at MD Anderson Cancer Center honoring Nobel laureate James Allison, whose research we had long supported. In the audience were dozens of grateful patients who, thanks to therapies developed by Jim, were in full remission from stage 4 melanoma diagnoses. A 2021 article in the *New England Journal of Medicine* said, "Treatment and survival for patients with . . . melanoma have improved dramatically in the past 10 years."

March on Washington, and new discoveries from genome sequencing. Greg made it a mission to link advocates for all life-threatening diseases in a combined cause. *FasterCures* soon became a trusted source of information and the global hub for more than a hundred disease-specific research groups. We spoke for many of these groups when we testified about pending legislation and brought members of Congress together with scientific leaders for the enlightenment of both.

Most importantly, *FasterCures* put patients first. One of our earliest programs was PHD—Patients Helping Doctors, which educated patients about the powerful role they can play. We began by encouraging these patients to enroll in clinical trials and urge their relatives to load their health metrics in data banks. It was part of the answer to loved ones who asked what they could do to help a desperately ill patient. It also provided real world evidence that helped clinicians better understand their patients' priorities.

Ever since the mid-1990s, we had helped create data and tissue consortiums across institutions. We'd gone on television urging patients to sign up for clinical trials and to donate data for family medical histories. If you're in the hospital, we told them, ask visiting relatives if they'd be willing to submit a DNA sample for research. All this was part of an effort to address the frustrations of researchers who lacked access to data on specific diseases. CaP CURE had shown what a highly focused disease-specific research organization could achieve. Now we sought to build research links *across* disease types. An early *FasterCures* publication "Think Research," showed the value of electronic medical records, not only as an efficiency tool, but also as a powerful means to aggregate data and accelerate medical solutions.

Among the experts and business executives Greg brought in to help him expand the *FasterCures* mission was Margaret Anderson.

Margaret had broad experience in biomedical and public health policy as well as deep knowledge of patient activism, which had begun with HIV/AIDS advocacy groups in the 1980s. After five years, Greg had an opportunity to move on to a very senior industry position and Margaret, who had been chief operating officer, succeeded him as executive director. She carried forward and enlarged *FasterCures* initiatives Greg had launched including the TRAIN network and the PHD program. Just as TRAIN allowed disease specific research organizations to learn best practices from each other, PHD helped doctors learn from their patients. Margaret dedicated herself to making *FasterCures* an even stronger hub by convening and connecting all parts of the medical research ecosystem. She also launched major new programs including Partnering for Cures (P4C).

A MATRIX APPROACH

By 2009, Margaret said it was time to bring all the players in the health infrastructure together in an annual meeting for hands-on problem-solving. Every year thereafter, a growing number of leaders from government, industry, patient groups, the investment community, foundations and academic medical centers convened for the *FasterCures* Partnering for Cures conference.

We took a matrix approach at P4C. Part of the agenda included an exchange of information on the latest medical technologies; and part was a program that brought disease-specific groups together to find common areas. P4C's speaker presentations and panels attracted large audiences and coverage by the national media. But the real value of this unique gathering was in the networking opportunities. In something akin to biomedical speed dating, nearly two hundred groups signed up for short get-acquainted chats with others who might share their research interests. We view these organizations as valuable partners in our own efforts to accelerate medical solutions.

The Milken Institute and *FasterCures* executives shared our extensive knowledge of the medical research process with philanthropists searching for ways to make their charitable giving more effective. Leading this effort was Melissa Stevens, deputy executive director of *FasterCures* and the head of its Philanthropy Advisory Service. Eventually, this activity became so extensive and its knowledge base so deep that PAS was elevated to become a standalone group—the Milken Institute Center for Strategic Philanthropy (CSP).

CSP works with individual philanthropists, families, and foundations seeking to deploy their capital to make a transformative, sustainable impact. Melissa had previously used her experience as a health sciences consultant at PricewaterhouseCoopers to advise commercial and federal clients. Over the past several years, she has overseen strategies that influenced more than one billion dollars in philanthropic giving.

In 2018, Partnering for Cures became the Milken Institute's annual Future of Health Summit and relocated from New York to Washington, where it's more convenient for members of Congress, cabinet secretaries, and other policy leaders.*

---

* Also in 2018, California governor Jerry Brown asked me to serve as the *FasterCures* representative on a governor's advisory committee on personalized medicine. Our mandate was to develop legislative proposals to accelerate clinical breakthroughs. Over the following year, we produced detailed recommendations that were submitted to the legislature. Part of our analysis was the observation that "personalized medicine" no longer adequately described the shift away from one-size-fits-all therapies. It had already become "precision medicine" because of advanced genome-sequencing capabilities. The ultimate goal was "precision health," which recognizes a more holistic approach to patient needs beyond initial treatment.

FIGHTING TREATMENT DISPARITIES

At one of our early P4C conferences, Margaret asked me to take a side meeting with someone I hadn't met previously. She assured me it would be a good use of my time. That's when I was introduced to Freda Lewis-Hall, MD. Only a handful of people have fundamentally altered the way I see the world—people who literally changed my life. One was the man I met on a street in the riot-torn Watts neighborhood of Los Angeles during the summer of 1965. Another was Jim Allison, who mobilized me to focus on immunology. A third influencer was Trip Casscells, whose example of courage and leadership in the face of adversity still inspires me.

Then there's Freda. Her passion for medicine and for patients was apparent from the very first time we sat down together in New York more than a decade ago. She changed my understanding of the ways many patients view biomedical research.

"My parents migrated from Richmond, Virginia, up to Maryland in 1945," she said, "because Richmond was a hard place to be a Black person in those days. My dad and his older brothers had grown up near a canning factory where they'd collect discarded corn cobs, dry them, and then sell them for cooking fires." That kind of industriousness must have rubbed off on Dr. Lewis-Hall because at age six she decided to become a physician. However, a school counselor said young Freda Lewis was "a lovely lady with good manners" who should marry well so she could be "a good wife to someone with a future." Freda's mother, whose education had ended with high school, was livid when she heard this and promptly brought home a stack of college guides. (A few years later, Freda did "marry well," but not so she could be a subservient spouse. She and the love of her life, Randy Hall, both had "a future"—they married while he was at Penn Law School and she was beginning medical training.)

After graduating from the Johns Hopkins University and Howard University Medical School, Freda trained in psychiatry. Her first job as a psychiatrist was in the US Virgin Islands where she was once threatened by a psychotic patient with a machete. That harrowing experience didn't deter her, but about that time another opportunity arose in the form of a job offer from pharmaceutical giant Eli Lilly. She had been concerned about the lack of information on treatment of mental disorders with psychoactive drugs—especially treatment of African Americans and women. The offer from Lilly would allow her to study a large database of information that might help these neglected patients.

When I met Freda, she had become executive vice president and chief medical officer at Pfizer. It was early December and as we chatted, she mentioned a recent Thanksgiving dinner with her extended family. Rather than congratulating her on ascending to one of the most prominent positions in the pharmaceutical industry, they told her they were disappointed that she worked on the "dark side" of healthcare: "You were always the smartest student in your school and we thought you had such promise as a doctor. We didn't expect you to sell out to one of those big corporations." Her father then excused himself to go take his Lipitor prescription, a statin made by Pfizer. Unknown to him, Freda's employer had developed his life-extending pill.

She received reassurance from her husband Randy: "You have always been a healer. Does it matter if it's one patient at a time or a million at a time?" She soon became a familiar face on television, appearing regularly on *The Doctors* and *Dr. Phil* as an advocate for patient-centered healthcare that works to reduce treatment disparities.*

---

* COVID-19 made these disparities painfully apparent: As of 2000, African Americans were 12 percent of the US population, but 33 percent of the pandemic's deaths; 17 percent of Americans are of Hispanic origin, but they have suffered 30 percent of deaths.

Like everyone involved in the medical research process, I've heard many of the crazy conspiracy theories about the supposed evils of Big Pharma that still circulate on social media. Freda told me she was in a taxi returning to her office at Pfizer's New York headquarters one afternoon when the driver told her he knew that the big drug companies had discovered the cure for cancer long ago. "They're keeping it a secret," he said, "because they make so much money off cancer patients." Freda doesn't let such nutty ideas discourage her. "It's a privilege and an honor to be part of an industry that focuses on patients, saves lives and advances science," she says.

By the way, her father continued to take his prescribed medications and lived to age one hundred.

OUR CONSISTENT MISSION

Freda now serves on the boards of *FasterCures*, the Prostate Cancer Foundation, and the Milken Institute. On the *FasterCures* advisory board, which includes three former FDA commissioners, she has been a strong supporter of our recent initiatives to link real-world patient data even more closely to the research process. Esther Krofah, a public policy expert, led development of this work from 2018 to 2020. As her new program was about to launch in March 2020, Esther was named *FasterCures's* executive director.

Within days of Esther's appointment, the COVID lockdown began and other plans were put on hold while all Milken Institute centers focused on the pandemic. Esther's previous work on data integration served her well as she and her staff launched a robust and effective response to the COVID challenge.

Looking back, it's clear that CaP CURE was really "*FasterCures*

1.0." *FasterCures* 2.0 included the expansion of our global programs across all diseases and institutions. Today's *FasterCures* is the 3.0 version—an international, data-driven organization that puts patients at the center of the research process and continues to disrupt the bottlenecks that slow the treatments they need.

EIGHTEEN

Innovate to Accelerate

Some people might have been distracted by the beauty of Lake Tahoe, glistening amid the splendor of the Sierra Nevada Basin. They were not part of the group we convened in July 2004 for the first *FasterCures* retreat. If the spectacular surroundings had an effect, it was only to inspire creativity. We had four days to tap the intellectual firepower of Nobel laureates, talented scientists, biotech entrepreneurs, foundation leaders, and business innovators. They would help *FasterCures* to sharpen its ambitious plans.

By the end of the twentieth century, more than one million Americans suffered heart attacks every year. Strokes hit 600,000. Cancer was killing 550,000. Alzheimer's, diabetes, kidney diseases, AIDS, and other serious conditions still devastated individuals and families. Medical scientists working on better treatments and cures faced a maze of conflicting incentives and often-outmoded regulations. We needed a more encompassing strategy for addressing these issues.

In preparation for the retreat, I had asked Caltech president and *FasterCures* board member David Baltimore to prepare some ideas for revolutionary change. As he put it, "We must undertake grand challenges if we want to reap the rewards of grand solutions." Other participants brought specific ideas for speeding the pace of discovery. One by one, they shared their goals, their insights and their frustrations.

Listening to them speak, I reflected on everything we'd done since 1993 to accelerate progress: call-to-action dinners; yearly scientific retreats; hundreds of Milken Institute Global Conference panels; white papers on nutrition and the microbiome; speeches; Young Investigator Awards; online information for patients and doctors; television appearances; magazine covers; the Home Run Challenge; the March on Washington; legislative initiatives; and more. We'd played a leadership role in the doubling of the NIH budget, supported centers of research excellence at academic institutions, recruited scientists, written healthy eating cookbooks, and talked constantly about the hope and promise of research. Still, I knew it wasn't enough.

A THREE-PART STRATEGY

Technology was advancing rapidly. In 2000, Francis Collins announced completion of the human genome's first draft. Francis was one of many scientists I consulted in developing a new strategy designed to bring the benefits of technology's advance to more patients. In a 2001 TED Talk, I advocated greater dedication to research acceleration and, for the first time, publicly disclosed plans for what would become *FasterCures*. Eventually, the outlines of a new strategy began to form. The strategy would focus our efforts in three areas:

1. Accelerate medical solutions, especially through greater data access.

2. Address the challenge of resources diverted to treat lifestyle diseases.

3. Generate more funding for research.

One of the first steps in implementing this strategy would be the separation of CaP CURE, which expanded into multiple organizations. In a 2003 article that accompanied the *FasterCures* launch, I told *Wall Street Journal* readers:

The choice is ours. We can sit back and wait for more cures and better treatments, or we can marshal our resources to solve problems sooner and save more lives. Maybe yours.

Expanding on that thought, I said to the retreat attendees, "Here's a simple request for each of you: Help us develop plans for an attack on disease that deploys the best resources of human capital, medical and biological information, and twenty-first-century technologies. Let's replace the old tracks that slow the train of progress."

In response, they worked out specific plans for better research collaboration, increased participation in clinical trials, improved data collection systems, new preclinical disease models, and more. These ideas built on the three-part strategy of acceleration, diversion avoidance and funding. They would be the basis of all *FasterCures* accomplishments over the next twenty years.

STRATEGY I—ACCELERATION

In December 2004, *FasterCures* brought together eighteen research funding organizations for a Summit on Innovation in Disease Research at Esquire House in Los Angeles. These groups helped us develop a comprehensive Innovation Agenda that included such components as research networks collaborating and exchanging case studies; new IT platforms and open source approaches; databanks of bio-specimens; and joint ventures among disease groups.

The next month, we held a forum at the Aspen Institute to expand the dialogue on how to integrate the needs of the clinical and biomedical research community into the development of the Bush Administration's proposed National Health Information Network. The Aspen discussions formed the basis for multiple panels at the 2005 Milken Institute Global Conference.

The day before the Global Conference opened to the public in Los Angeles, we hosted an all-day meeting—"New Approaches for New Outcomes"—at the Getty Center. Our invitation explained the *FasterCures* vision:

> *Imagine a future in which the journey from scientific discovery to clinical application takes a few years versus several decades. Envision a medical research community that collaborates—through sharing data and experience—to uncover radical new cures for deadly diseases.*

Among the many panelists were: Lee Hartwell, Nobel laureate and president of the Fred Hutchinson Cancer Research Center; William Haseltine, CEO of Human Genome Sciences; Kathy Giusti, president of the Multiple Myeloma Research Alliance; Lee Hood, president of the Institute for Systems Biology; Anna Barker, deputy director of the National Cancer Institute; and Craig Venter, founder of the Institute for Genomic Research.

The next three days at the Global Conference featured nearly twenty *FasterCures* panels with such titles as "Transforming Medicine from Reactive to Predictive to Preventive," "The Innovation Pipeline Race," "The Impact of Women's Health on the Global

Economy," "Designing a Twenty-First-Century Drug Approval System," "Medicine in Twenty Years," and "Financial Innovations to Spur Medical Research."

FasterCures continued a rapid pace of conferences, forums and summits seemingly every month including each year's Global Conference. Their work increased research collaborations while gaining increased notice by the media and by Washington policy leaders. Still, after several years, we began to sense that the most optimistic hopes for patient benefits from the human genome project and other programs remained largely unfulfilled. The field needed a reboot. We were especially focused on accelerating the process of turning basic science discoveries into practical therapies.

In September 2011, we convened a private weekend meeting for seventy of the most senior leaders from around the world on the shores of Lake Tahoe—the same location where the *FasterCures* strategy had been launched at the 2004 retreat. Chris Viehbacher, then the CEO of the pharmaceutical company Sanofi, and an outspoken champion of innovation, joined me in cohosting the event. As Chris and I told the attendees, "We're here to shake things up." The group included major corporate CEOs, members of Congress, medical school deans, federal agency directors, industry analysts, renowned scientists, and venture capitalists. Although our focus was bioscience, we included nonscientists and risk-takers in other fields. For example, Peter Ueberroth, once Time Man of the Year who had produced the successful 1984 Olympic Games, contributed valuable insights. As someone who knows how to get things done, Peter helped us explore the question of how to "innovate innovation" in medical research.

We asked everyone to read white papers in advance and to arrive ready to set a new health agenda for the country. I'd been curating the event for months to assure an eclectic group with the authority, knowledge, and willingness to drive change.

This event, the Lake Tahoe Retreat on Bioscience Innovation, was one of the most productive experiences of my long career. We referred to it as "forty-four hours to change the world." Discussions were frank, often heated, and grounded in reality. What emerged was a broad consensus on the priorities for public policy. The group recognized that innovations in bioscience would help shape the twenty-first century in areas that extend far beyond healthcare. These include:

+ Abundant food and clean water;

+ Shields against bioterrorism;

+ Reliable energy supplies;

+ National defense;

+ Protection from pandemics; and

+ Environmental sustainability.

Following the Retreat, *FasterCures* and others carried the message about translational science to policy makers on both sides of the aisle in Washington. We strongly supported proposed legislation that would create a new NIH organization, the National Center for Advancing Translational Sciences (NCATS).

Like the doubling of the NIH budget more than a decade earlier, the creation of NCATS would be a major step forward for the medical research process. The way we arrived there, however, was very different. Anyone who has created a household budget at the kitchen table understands the concept of government spending. That's why we created a "people's army"—hundreds of thousands strong—to march on Washington in 1998. The subsequent increase in NIH resources supported a crucial expansion of the agency's grant-making programs. Conversely, few people understand translational research and NCATS remains little known by the public despite its central role in speeding new therapies to patients. It would take an alternative strategy to include this proposed new institute in the Consolidated Appropriations Act of 2012.

All citizens are free to contact members of Congress to express opinions about pending legislation. But federal regulations prohibited agency heads like the NIH director from calling a senator to explain even the most complex proposals. NIH needed some help. Knowing that Harry Reid, the Democratic Senate Majority Leader, and Eric Cantor, the Republican House Majority Leader, were believers in the NCATS concept, I met with them and suggested they consider making it a priority during the fall session of Congress in 2011. They convinced many of their colleagues and Congress soon included NCATS in legislation signed by President Obama a few months later.

NCATS focuses on the fact that for every new drug or device approved by the FDA, hundreds of others fall by the wayside over five to fifteen years on the way from the laboratory to the patient. NCATS has been particularly effective in shortening and bridging this "valley of death" across the dozens of difficult steps needed to "translate" basic science into useful therapies. By analyzing similarities across several diseases, NCATS has helped develop multiple treatments in less time; and in doing this, they've developed models that better predict a patient's reaction to treatment.

Never has this process been more valuable than during the COVID-19 crisis. NCATS was at the center of the NIH response: It made sure that the agency had optimized the screening of all existing compounds that might be active against the virus; it coordinated the efforts of some sixty institutions that were planning clinical trials; and then it convinced them to contribute their clinical data. This showed what the virus was doing to patients and how those patients responded to different treatments. In hindsight, this might seem obvious; but it took bold leadership and diplomatic skill for a federal agency to pull it off.*

STRATEGY II—ADDRESSING RESOURCE DIVERSION

We had entered the new century with confidence that Americans would enjoy better health built on the march of medical progress. It seemed obvious that the leading nations throughout the century would be those that remained preeminent in bioscience. The United States had been a fount of innovation for decades and seemed destined to continue that leadership. Unfortunately, however, many of our most talented physicians and medical scientists were being diverted to deal with the growing burden of chronic diseases. One of the biggest contributors to that burden was an epidemic of obesity. Significant resources had to be dedicated to treating the consequences of lifestyle-related disease—resources drawn from basic, translational and clinical research. It was a public health crisis.

I used various approaches in my speeches, sometimes displaying shocking statistics about the tragic burden of disease. On other occasions, my presentation would include humorous cartoons and videos. It wasn't hard to make the audiences laugh. The hard part was getting them to change their habits.

---

* The director of NCATS through its first decade was Christopher Austin, MD, a delightfully irrepressible public servant. Chris almost didn't pursue a medical career. A gifted opera singer, he faced a difficult choice during his college years: pursue an apparently bright future as a professional vocalist or go to medical school. Although he chose medicine, he never entirely forsook singing. On several occasions when he joined us at Milken Institute events, I convinced him to entertain the audience with a thrilling rendition of a Mozart or Verdi aria. After nineteen years of service at the NIH, Chris returned to private industry in 2021.

Another approach involved teaming up with corporate leaders who shared our concern about destructive lifestyle habits. The healthcare costs for American companies were rising rapidly. Firms such as Safeway developed insurance plans that provided incentives for employees that could substantially reduce their health insurance premiums by reducing weight, cholesterol, blood pressure and tobacco usage.

UNHEALTHY AMERICA

Several Global Conference panels over the years focused on the idea that the right foods can help prevent chronic diseases. We conducted our own research and published the findings in the Milken Institute report, *An Unhealthy America: The Economic Burden of Chronic Disease (2007)*. Among the report's findings:

+ More than half of Americans suffer from one or more chronic diseases. The seven most common are cancer, diabetes, hypertension, stroke, heart disease, pulmonary conditions, and mental disorders.

+ Obesity contributes to all of these chronic conditions. Just the change in the population's average weight over fifteen years cost the US more than $1 trillion annually.

+ Much of the cost is avoidable through prevention.

In the years following that seminal publication, other Institute studies dealt with prevention and wellness, aging, and American leadership in bioscience. In 2018, a new Milken Institute report— *The Costs of Chronic Disease in the United States*—broke down the direct, indirect and total costs of twenty-four chronic diseases. Indirect costs include work absences, lost wages, and reduced productivity.

The total bill was $3.7 trillion a year, much of it preventable. It noted that the aging of the US population would significantly increase these costs absent some effective interventions.

Unhealthy America and later reports helped increase public awareness of lifestyle issues. We had defined the nation's health challenges dramatically and shown what actions could make people healthier and the economy more productive. Feeling that we were gaining traction, we turned to the next challenge. The third part of our overall strategy was to get the America's leaders behind the idea of a national rededication to bioscience and to put dollars behind that idea by resuming NIH budget increases.

STRATEGY III—FUNDING RESEARCH

Given all the political rancor about healthcare legislation in 2012, another massive demonstration like our 1998 March wouldn't work. But we had a plan that was based in part on our success in helping get NCATS approved. It involved a carefully orchestrated event—a Celebration of Science—focused on about a thousand senior leaders. That event, spanning the weekend after Labor Day 2012, was devoted to a single proposition: Science matters. We intended to highlight the economic and social benefits of scientific research, encourage students to pursue careers in the biological sciences, engage the nation's political leadership as active participants, and build a groundswell of support for renewed commitments from government, industry and philanthropies.

Over three days, the Celebration of Science convened the leaders of the US House and Senate from both parties with scientists, university presidents, corporate CEOs, cabinet secretaries, philanthropists, and patient advocates. The opening sessions at the George Washington University included basketball legend and HIV/AIDS spokesman Magic Johnson and Dr. Anthony Fauci, director of the NIH National Institute of Allergy and Infectious Diseases. I remember the stark contrast between the five-foot-six Tony Fauci and the six-foot-nine Johnson.

We included Magic—an athlete, not a scientist—in this scientific event because he symbolized something very important. Back in 1987, popular TV host Oprah Winfrey had opened an afternoon broadcast with this shocking prediction:

> *Hello, everybody. AIDS has both sexes running scared. Research studies now project that one in five-listen to me, hard to believe-one in five heterosexuals could be dead from AIDS at the end of the next three years. That's by 1990. One in five. It is no longer just a gay disease.*

In 1991, just four years later, Magic held an emotional press conference announcing his retirement from basketball. At the time, he had tested positive for the AIDS virus. Most people thought he was dying. He thought he was dying. At the time, some players shunned him, even refusing to shake hands. It reminded me of the early 1950s when parents told their children not to use public water fountains because they might catch polio.

Magic later told an interviewer that his good friend (and on-court rival) Larry Bird called him as soon as he heard the news:

> *We were talking, it's just, "How you doin'? Heard about it." You can almost hear both of us with some tears in our eyes. And I'm choked up because he did call me. When something happens to you and then you find out who really your friends are and people who really care about you.*

Thanks to antiretroviral therapy, Magic did not die—and here he was in 2012, bigger than life, with a mile-wide smile. It helped us make the point that science can triumph over disease, and it did so far more powerfully than any statistical report.

MIND BLOWING

For many years, one of the most popular Milken Institute Global Conference panels has been called "Things That Will Blow Your Mind." That evening during the Celebration of Science, we gathered at the National Portrait Gallery for a dinner that included presentations on future technologies. Later, retired Army General Peter Chiarelli, a leader in national mental health programs, discussed advances using technology to treat our wounded warriors. Then he introduced a special guest, retired captain Dan Berschinski. Some in the audience gasped as Dan gamely negotiated three steps up to the stage on his two prosthetic legs. Despite his injuries, he told us that he was one of the lucky ones who remained whole—in spirit if not in body. Many veterans, he said, may look healthy, but suffer from deep psychological scars.

The next morning, NIH Director Francis Collins welcomed nearly a thousand of us to that agency's Bethesda headquarters. It was huge logistic challenge to move such a large crowd quickly through NIH security. All went smoothly and our group appreciated a day of presentations highlighting the incredible diversity and benefits of NIH-sponsored research. We saw stunning technological advances that might lead to future cures. Everyone at the NIH was very proud that their achievements were being highlighted for us by their leader.

The NIH supports research in hundreds of areas. We asked Francis to focus on a few with the most emotional impact. This included stories told by patients: fatally ill children restored to full enjoyment of life; a breakthrough treatment providing the gift of breath for cystic fibrosis sufferers; new drugs that allowed an HIV-positive woman to give birth to healthy children; and much more.

I will never forget the presentation of Dawn Averitt Bridge, a remarkable woman who founded the AIDS Survival Project and served on the Presidential Advisory Committee on HIV/AIDS. Dawn was diagnosed with HIV in 1988 at age nineteen after being raped while working in Spain. She had always hoped to have children, but at the time, about 98 percent of babies born to HIV-positive mothers inherited the virus. However, thanks to NIH-sponsored research, new HIV therapies eventually made it possible for nearly all such mothers to deliver a child safely. In my mind, I can still see the photograph of Dawn's beautiful first baby projected on the screen behind her.

Then there was a wounded soldier—a double amputee—who, thanks to implanted brain sensors, could now pick up a glass with his prosthetic right arm just by thinking about the maneuver. His grateful wife was in tears, and so were many of us watching. It was impressive, especially to the several members of Congress in the audience.

That night, we moved to the Kennedy Center for the Performing Arts where an eclectic combination of senior government leaders, scientists, musicians, and entertainers became part of a memorable event. Speakers included Senate Majority Leader Harry Reid, House Majority Leader Eric Cantor, and House Minority Leader Nancy Pelosi as well as several other members of Congress. In an extraordinary outpouring of bipartisan commitment, they pledged to work across the aisle in support of science.

The first few rows were reserved for dozens of our Young Investigators who were working to advance medical science. Our message to them was that they had chosen the right career and the nation appreciated it. Everything about the evening was designed to convince the congressional leadership to increase federal support for health agencies. All the events we had sponsored since the mid-1990s were planned to help rededicate America to bioscience. But Washington is a skeptical town and we needed to make a powerful case for that cause.

Hosts Whoopi Goldberg and John O'Hurley introduced videos about progress against disease interspersed with brief talks by members of Congress and leading scientists. It was to be the last public appearance by US Senator Daniel Inouye, a military hero who served in public office for fifty-eight years. We recognized his many legislative achievements that included strong support for healthcare. Sitting near Senator Inouye was the widow of the late Senator Ted Stevens, who had participated in our Scientific Retreats at Lake Tahoe and played a crucial role in passage of the legislation establishing the Department of Defense cancer research program.

Many in the audience related to a video showing the burdens shouldered by caretakers of Alzheimer's disease patients. After we played a particularly emotional short movie of children with cystic fibrosis, there wasn't a dry eye in the audience.* Whoopi was so moved by seeing these kids struggling to breathe that she announced she was giving up smoking cigarettes immediately.

THE ROCK DOCS

Then it was time for what the program called the Entertainers of Science. But most of us referred to them as the Rock Docs. It turns out that many great medical researchers are accomplished musicians. Among the physicians and scientists led by NIH Director Francis Collins that night were four keyboard players, five guitarists, one singing bass player, one drummer, one flute player, two trumpeters,

---

* With the latest drugs for CS, more than eighty percent of these children can now enjoy nearly normal lives.

a saxophonist and one lone harmonica player (who happened to be future Nobel laureate Jim Allison). Their performances of "You've Got a Friend," "Here Comes the Sun," and "Help!" had the audience on its feet. It showed that these great scientists were not some kind of icons on a pedestal, but really dedicated human beings who happened to enjoy music and entertaining.

A little later, ten-time Grammy winner Kenny (Babyface) Edmonds, took the stage. He was to perform a musical tribute to his late father, who died from lung cancer. But no one had told him he was scheduled to play after the Rock Docs. "That was completely unfair," he said with a sly smile. Then he added, "Maybe I should go to medical school." Other musical performances included Grammy winner Melissa Manchester, who dedicated her hit song "Don't Cry Out Loud" to wounded veterans, and singer Stevie Nicks, formerly of Fleetwood Mac, who had often visited injured soldiers at Walter Reed Army Medical Center.

The three-day event concluded with more panels at George Washington University that included Nobel laureate James Watson, Energy Secretary Steven Chu, White House science advisor John Holdren and several other internationally known scientists.

The Celebration of Science went a long way toward raising the profile of America's bioscience achievements. In the years since, Congress once again started increasing NIH funding. Overall, in the quarter century since our 1998 March on Washington, they have provided approximately $500 billion in incremental resources for NIH-sponsored research.

Each of three events—the March on Washington, the Retreat on Bioscience Innovation at Lake Tahoe, and the Celebration of Science in Washington—was implemented with a specific strategy. The combined cost of the three events was no more than $15 to 20 million. That investment has paid off thousands of times over.

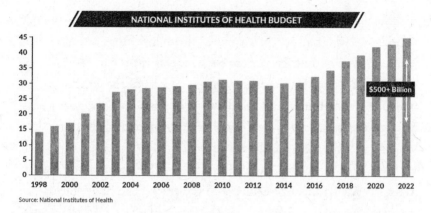

NATIONAL INSTITUTES OF HEALTH BUDGET

$500+ Billion

Source: National Institutes of Health

CURES

Less than two years after the Celebration of Science, a bipartisan coalition in the House and Senate proposed what became the 21st Century Cures Act. I testified in support of the Act before the House Energy and Commerce Committee. For another two years we worked closely with the committee's then-chairman, Republican Fred Upton, and ranking member, Democrat Diana DeGette. The Cures Act had provisions aimed at breaking down interdisciplinary and inter-institutional silos; restructuring parts of the FDA and streamlining its drug-approval process; and providing $6.3 billion for new initiatives in precision medicine, studies of the brain, cancer and regenerative medicine.*

In late 2016, we hosted a private dinner at the Jefferson Hotel, a few blocks up Sixteenth Street from the White House. The dozen or so guests included Tennessee Senator Lamar Alexander, the head of

---

* It just happened that one section of the act—little noticed at the time—gave the NIH important operational flexibility when the coronavirus crisis began. In April 2020, Congress quickly provided $1.5 billion to the NIH under the "Other Transaction Authority" of the Cures Act. This funded a crucial new initiative called RADX—Rapid Acceleration of Diagnostics.

the Senate health committee; NIH Director Francis Collins; Peggy Hamburg, who had recently stepped down as FDA Commissioner; and some senior executives from large biopharmaceutical companies. Knowing that there were widely varying views of the Cures Act, we scheduled this dinner for a frank airing of positions. The goal was to provide a safe, off-the-record environment where these leaders could express their thoughts and frustrations.

Sometime after the initial pleasantries, the discussion grew intense. Peggy had mentioned several reforms at the FDA during her tenure. One of the pharma CEOs then jumped in to ask her what she ever did for his industry. He claimed the FDA just slowed things down by preventing new drugs from coming to market. At that point, Senator Alexander, known as a consensus builder, smoothed things over by noting some of the benefits for drug companies in the proposed legislation.

As voting on the act approached, I wrote an op-ed article in the *Wall Street Journal* urging Congress to pass it. I can't claim credit—many other individuals and organizations were behind the effort—but in a coincidence of timing, the day after my article appeared, the House of Representatives voted in favor of the Act by the overwhelmingly positive margin of 392–26. Later, the Senate passed the bill 94–5. President Obama signed the law at the end of 2016.

Four years after the 21st Century Cures Act became law, Representatives Upton and DeGette participated in the Milken Institute's 2020 Future of Health Summit. That very day, the FDA had given final approval to the first COVID-19 vaccine. Congressman Upton wrote in his next constituent newsletter that the Cures Act "shaved many months—perhaps years—off what would have been the approval process for a COVID vaccine."

In 2021, the bipartisan Upton-DeGette team introduced follow-on legislation that called for establishment of a new DARPA-like agency—the Advanced Research Projects Agency for Health

(ARPA-H). I wrote another article calling ARPA-H "the next step toward faster cures."* Then in February 2022, *FasterCures* Executive Director Esther Krofah testified before a House subcommittee in support of the new agency. A month later, Congress passed a spending bill that included $1 billion for ARPA-H, which has now begun operations with a high degree of flexibility to pursue high-risk, high-reward disease research.

It's been twenty years since we launched the new strategy based on defining the nation's health challenges, demonstrating what could work, creating a plan of action; convening the right people to implement it, and seeing it through to legislative success. The *FasterCures* team has done a great job of refocusing our country on medical research. In recent years, they've also expanded our work on the other major component of the national health infrastructure—public health.

---

* See my July 27, 2021, *Wall Street Journal* op-ed, "COVID Is the 21st Century's Sputnik" at www.mikemilken.com.

NINETEEN

Public Health

On a cold January day in 2014, Atlanta nearly ground to a halt. The city, which rarely experiences severe winter weather, was buffeted by ice, sleet, and intermittent snow flurries. Hundreds of flights were canceled and driving became treacherous. The timing couldn't have been worse because we'd invited 300 health leaders from across the country to join us the next morning at the US Centers for Disease Control and Prevention. How many would make it?

The agency had never before agreed to open its world-renowned laboratories and offices to this kind of group. Security was tight—CDC headquarters includes a Biosafety Level-4 laboratory housing some of the world's most dangerous microbes. We'd been planning for months. Georgia Governor Nathan Deal and US Senator Johnny Isakson would kick things off before a series of all-star panels. There'd be a tour of the Emergency Operations Center, a massive room that looked like NASA's Mission Control where scientists tracked disease outbreaks anywhere on the planet. The day would end with a tour of the CDC Museum.

Almost all our guests managed to get there. Some even drove hundreds of miles after their flights were diverted to other cities. The Summit participants represented what could have been considered a board of directors of American public health. Even then, six years before the first COVID-19 lockdowns, we knew that an infectious disease pandemic was a very real threat. The day's panels included:

- ♦ Global Health Security: Containing Threats Worldwide
- ♦ Outsmarting Superbugs: A Race We Can't Afford to Lose
- ♦ The Business Case for Public Health

We worked with the CDC Foundation to convene this unique event—the Summit on Public Health and Prosperity—as part of our strategy for addressing health threats and the chronic diseases that divert talent away from medical research.

Between the last panel and an evening reception, a group of us walked through museum exhibits. As others moved on, I watched a

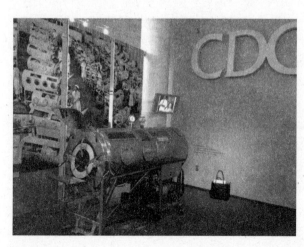

This iron lung at CDC head-quarters evoked poignant memories of my father's polio.

254 | FASTER CURES

decades-old film of a man lying in an iron lung, a machine that created pressure to expand and contract the lungs of polio patients no longer able to breathe on their own. Every few seconds, an artificial diaphragm made a *whoosh, whoosh* sound as it moved in and out.

It was difficult to watch this unfortunate patient whose inert body was trapped inside a metal chamber with only his head visible. Surprisingly, he seemed happy, even jovial. After many years in his sad position, he had accepted fate and adapted. He read books, watched TV and chatted with friends on the phone.

Behind the display of an actual machine, a 1950s photograph showed an "iron lung hotel" where nurses tended to patients secured inside dozens of the devices.

SALK, SMALLPOX, AND SAFETY

Polio was an immediate threat for those of us who grew up in the 1950s. I recall one morning in 1955 when we lined up to get jabbed with a needle at Hesby Street School. I'd read about polio and understood that the Salk vaccine we received was part of a great public health victory. Yet even today, many people don't realize what the term "public health" means. Some think it's like public housing—a government welfare program. Others confuse it with health insurance or medical research. Perhaps that's why it gets such short shrift in America. According to Atul Gawande, the surgeon and author, we spend about $12,000 a year per capita on medical treatments and a mere $56 on state and local public health departments. It doesn't seem to have occurred to most people that more spending on the latter could reduce the former.

Public health programs—including basic sanitation, vaccination campaigns, seat belt laws, occupational safety, air quality improvement, tobacco control, and nutrition education—have saved far more lives than all medical/surgical interventions combined. Dr. Leana Wen, a professor at the Milken Institute School of Public Health at George Washington University, likes to quote an old saying: "Public health saved your life today; you just don't know it." Or as Dr. William Foege, who devised the strategy that eliminated smallpox puts it, "Nobody ever thanks you for saving them from the disease they didn't know they were going to get."

The practice of medicine is different from public health. Physicians are trained in biological sciences, physiology, pharmacology, genomics, and related areas to diagnose and treat disease in individual patients. Most are not extensively trained in the specialized skills of public health—behavioral science, biostatistics, epidemiology, environmental health, demography and health services administration. A surgeon can remove a tumor from your lung; a public health practitioner focuses on the pollution and patterns of smoking that put the lungs of entire populations at risk. Doctors treat injuries caused by unsafe products; public health sets safety standards to prevent such accidents.

INCREASED FOCUS

Our focus on public health began long before the Atlanta Summit. CaP CURE had emphasized nutrition as a public health concern from its earliest days in the 1990s. It was part of the *FasterCures* mission when we launched that Milken Institute center in 2003. In 2007, we had published *An Unhealthy America*. The 2011 Lake Tahoe Retreat on Bioscience Innovation included an economic analysis of chronic diseases. That analysis convinced me that we had to be more active in addressing the complementary needs of both medical research and public health. Each would be more effective if we treated them as undivided parts of a broad health strategy.

As our focus on public health continued to grow, I realized that America's schools of public health were underfunded compared to professional graduate schools in other fields. Their alumni often had less capability to make major gifts. This was a cause for concern since our research showed that about 70 percent of healthcare costs relate to diseases linked to lifestyle. We began to explore ways the Milken Institute could help lift the importance of the public health profession and the careers of its practitioners.

This led us to George Washington University's program. GWU's public health school was literally at the center of the public health universe, a short walk from the White House, the State Department, the World Bank, Red Cross, and International Monetary Fund. It's a short taxi ride to Congress, the National Academies, the Health and Human Services Department, the AMA, the CDC's Washington office, and the American Cancer Society. Cross the Potomac River and you're at the National Science Foundation and the Pentagon. In the other direction, just inside Maryland, are the FDA and the National Institutes of Health. In other words, all the key health decision makers at the national level. Obviously, GW had an ideal physical location; now we wanted to be sure they had enough leadership talent.

The public health dean, Dr. Lynn Goldman, was highly regarded in the field. A physician, epidemiologist, and environmental health specialist, she had previously directed the Environmental Protection Agency's toxic substances division. Her effective work in that and other roles had earned her many awards for keeping dangerous chemicals and pesticides out of the environment.

About that time, we were also planning the 2012 Celebration of Science. Since the event would involve the NIH and other Washington-based agencies, it occurred to me that asking GW's public health school to host several of the panels would be a good test of their management skill. We also invited presidents of other leading universities to participate in the panels so we could gauge the respect they afforded GW. The events were a great success and encouraged us to begin a series of discussions about a more substantial GW-Milken Institute relationship.

The next year, as the discussions with GW continued, Dr. Thomas Frieden, director of the Centers for Disease Control and Prevention, spoke at the Milken Institute Global Conference to raise awareness of public health issues. I was impressed with Tom's Global Conference presentation and later invited him to join me on a panel at GW. He lamented the widespread public misunderstanding of public health in general and the CDC's role in particular. I suggested we could address that problem by bringing a high-level group of health leaders to the CDC's Atlanta headquarters. Tom quickly agreed and offered to host and help organize the Summit on Public Health.

PUBLIC HEALTH LEADERSHIP

Soon after that 2014 public health conference, GW announced gifts totaling $80 million to address public health challenges, especially disease prevention and wellness promotion. The contributions came from the Milken Institute, the Sumner M. Redstone Charitable Foundation and the Milken Family Foundation. In recognition of these gifts, the GW board of trustees announced the naming of the Milken Institute School of Public Health (MISPH). As part of the MISPH announcement, Lori and I created an endowed chair for the dean of the school as well as a new public health scholarship program. In the years since, we've made substantial additional contributions.

The late Sumner Redstone, whose business I had financed, had many debates and discussions with me about the value of nutrition. Originally a skeptic, he eventually became a strong advocate for healthy eating. This led to the Redstone Foundation's gift to the MISPH, which helped establish the school's Global Center for Prevention and Wellness. We recruited Dr. William Dietz, one of America's foremost authorities on obesity, to lead this new center.

Under Lynn Goldman's leadership, and with an expanded endowment, the MISPH has nearly tripled its enrollment to more than 3,200 students—the next generation of national and global public health leaders.

In 2022, *Fortune* magazine named it the nation's best online graduate program in public health. Its leadership role is confirmed by the fact that Lynn and other members of its faculty are interviewed almost daily for articles in the national media related to the COVID pandemic and other public health matters. Lynn's peers in the Association of Schools and Programs in Public Health, representing more than a hundred institutions, recently elected her as chair of its board of directors.

Separate from the MISPH, we established the Milken Institute Center for Public Health as a research and program hub for all the schools and programs in public health across North America. The center cohosts the annual Future of Health Summit and pursues programs related to mental health, food insecurity, the opioid crisis, isolation of seniors, obesity, disaster recovery, healthcare affordability, and the widespread impacts of COVID-19.

OUTRUNNING THE ENEMY

Despite the worldwide doubling of life expectancy in a single century, much remains to be done. A 2019 Milken Institute Review article cited a Global Burden of Disease study listing the top five risk factors for premature death: dietary risks; high systolic blood pressure, tobacco, high fasting-plasma glucose (poorly controlled diabetes), and air pollution. One or more Milken Institute centers is working on each of these challenges.

Behavioral issues such as obesity, smoking, gun violence, and opioid use impose a real social cost. Yet there's often vehement disagreement about proposed cures. Most people don't want to be taxed or lectured to. So we all bear the burden. There are no simple solutions.

It would help if we gave public health professionals better pay and program support. We need them not just to prepare for the next viral pandemic, but also to deal with antibiotic-resistant superbugs—the bacterial enemies that could devastate our society. We need them in all health sectors—private nonprofit organizations, industry and government; we need all these sectors working together; and we need a sustained commitment, not just a crisis response. This is especially important in responding to the needs of underserved communities where the level of trust in the health system is often lower.

VETERANS DESERVE THE BEST

In 2016, we built on the success of our research template to launch one of the most significant public health initiatives of the last several years. The US Department of Veterans Affairs (VA) and the Prostate Cancer Foundation announced a $50 million public-private partnership to deliver precision oncology—the highest standard of care—to all veterans battling cancer. The VA already housed one of the world's largest health databases and this program effectively doubled its cancer research portfolio.

The partnership is establishing multiple PCF-VA Centers of Excellence (CoEs) across the nation. These centers advance cutting-edge medical research, deliver new genomic treatments, and provide a road map to apply precision medicine solutions for all forms of cancer and other life-threatening diseases. Any veteran entering a CoE now has access not only to the local VA hospital, but also to the resources of a leading nongovernmental medical center in the area.

The PCF-VA partnership is also training a cadre of precision oncology physicians and advanced-practice "data nurses of the future" who have specialized expertise in data management and clinical trial design. It's the first coordinated national network for multiple clinical trials.* The results of our partnership to date have been remarkable. We're getting close to achieving our goal of giving every veteran the highest quality of care—the same care our most fortunate private citizens would receive at any leading cancer center, as well as the same access to genomics research and clinical trials.

Precision oncology is one of the keys to ending deaths from cancer. By sequencing the genes in a patient's tumor, doctors can create a custom-tailored treatment plan that targets a cancer by its unique biology and genetic signature. And given the VA's leadership in telemedicine, advances from our program will be scalable and available anywhere. The PCF was the first mover in working with the VA. Now, other disease-focused organizations—including those dealing with cancers of the breast, lungs, and pancreas—are adopting similar VA partnerships. This is one more example of building on the template we first created in 1993—fund the initial model in one disease and if it's successful, deploy it in others.

---

* We were about to launch a series of cancer clinical trials across this network when the coronavirus struck. Fortunately, we had an infrastructure in place and could immediately redeploy our teams to confront the public health emergency. We moved quickly to establish the approved protocols for COVID-19 clinical trials of existing treatments that had been developed with PCF support. One such trial involved the same type of prostate cancer drugs to suppress testosterone that I had been taking for twenty-seven years. Various reports suggested that these drugs block the uptake of the COVID-19 virus by a co-receptor in the lungs. The virus depends on a protein called TMPRSS2, which is also found in prostate cancer and which needs testosterone to have its damaging effects.

A UNIQUE SUBPOPULATION

Dr. Richard Stone, the executive in charge of the VA's Veterans Health Administration, reports that African American men have a much lower prostate cancer survival rate than all other racial or ethnic groups—*except in one subpopulation*: veterans in the VA.* "We think that is a testament to the [PCF-VA] partnership," Dr. Stone told me.

A final thought about veterans. Those who have served in the military sometimes isolate themselves and experience intense loneliness. If you know any of these heroes, consider making a phone call just to say you're thinking about them, that you wish them well, and that you're interested in what's going on in their lives.

---

* In the general population, African Americans are 64 percent more likely to develop prostate cancer compared to any other race or ethnicity and 2.4 times more likely to die from the disease. Part of this disparity is rooted in biology; but the greatest impact is from access to care. See "How PCF Is Furthering Health Equity" at www.pcf.org.

PART IV

Priorities for the Future

TWENTY

COVID and Its Lessons

———————

Taking off from Tambo International Airport, we circle once above Johannesburg and rise quickly over the Witwatersrand range, out beyond the countless suburbs, up through the clouds to level off in the pure stillness of an African night. We're heading home.

Southern California is twenty hours away. Time to think and plan, as I always do on a long flight. Yet this trip is different: a crisis is coming.

Only a month earlier, just days after health officials from Wuhan, China, released the genetic sequence of a novel coronavirus, Nobel laureate David Baltimore had been in our Santa Monica offices. He came to record a video for an unrelated project. But we wanted to know what the famed virologist made of a still-small news item about a pneumonia outbreak half a world away. At that point, only a few hundred people had been infected in China and a handful had died. David has been a close friend for thirty-five years, long before he was president of Caltech, and he's never pulled punches. "Watch this one closely," he warned. "It's not likely to stay in China."

Still, with only some isolated cases, our planning for a twelve-day mission to nine cities in five countries continued.

The itinerary included the Milken Institute's annual Middle East and Africa Summit in Abu Dhabi. This popular event was overbooked with one telling exception: the delegation from China had just canceled.

EXTRA PRECAUTIONS

At that point, no cases had been reported in Africa and no one saw the need for personal protective equipment. Still, I loaded our plane with a supply of masks and disinfectant wipes, even pulling out an old wrist guard I'd used years earlier after breaking my wrist. Wearing the guard could prevent any social awkwardness if I declined to shake hands.

The first stop in the Middle East was Riyadh, where we met with the leadership of Saudi Arabia's B20, the business adjunct to the G20 nations. Next was a short hop to the United Arab Emirates for the Middle East and Africa Summit in Abu Dhabi. After the summit, we made a brief stop in Bahrain to participate in a one-day Investcorp seminar on economic development and health. At each of these venues, I spoke about the healthcare needs of Africa's growing populations and the effectiveness of the free enterprise system in providing economic opportunities across the continent.

Our seven-hour flight south to Johannesburg provided an opportunity to catch up on emails and international news reports. Global awareness of the COVID-19 threat was starting to grow. Italy had suspended flights to China and declared a national emergency. Still, South Africa appeared to be free of this disease, and we didn't break out the masks.

I looked forward to the coming events hosted by Patrice Motsepe and his wife Dr. Precious Moloi-Motsepe.* The Motsepe Foundation and the Prostate Cancer Foundation had been collaborating with the South African minister of health and the South Africa Medical Association to create a national strategic plan for cancer care and research. They had invited dozens of the nation's health leaders to a Johannesburg workshop, one of many PCF programs designed to extend its US-based research progress around the world.

During the return flight to Los Angeles, the subject lines in my email inbox spoke of growing global alarm about the World Health Organization's latest announcement. They had upgraded the coronavirus situation from a "technical concern" to a public health emergency. I needed to think it through.

It looks like it's going to be a health crisis of epic proportions. It will also be an economic disaster. What can we do that might have a chance to change the course of this disease?

As we headed west toward home, I reviewed the strengths of our medical foundations, the Milken Institute's centers around the world, and the Milken Institute School of Public Health. Then I sent messages to the leaders of these organizations to be ready for a COVID-19 planning meeting as soon as possible.

---

* Patrice and Precious have joined me in creating the Milken-Motsepe Prize. Among the first to address COVID-19 in South Africa, they pledged $55 million to the cause. Ironically, under the old apartheid regime, Precious—now the Chancellor of the University of Cape Town—would not have been permitted to attend that university.

RESEARCH AT BREAKNECK SPEED

In the first week of March, I flew up to meet with David Feinberg, who was then the head of Google Health at the company's Mountain View, California, headquarters. The billions of daily searches on Google could become a valuable epidemiological asset in tracing the path of disease.

On March 11, the World Health Organization labeled COVID-19 a pandemic. Within a few days, the structure of daily life turned upside down—businesses and schools closed, entertainment venues canceled productions, professional baseball and basketball teams stopped playing . . . and we all started wearing masks. Terms like "flattening the curve" and "cytokine storm" became part of daily news reports. Stock of a previously little-known company called Zoom Video Communications zoomed skyward. More ominously, cases of COVID followed a similar upward track. Hospitals were soon overwhelmed.

By the third week in March, COVID was killing fifteen hundred people every day around the world. On April 1, that quadrupled to more than six thousand.* I told my colleagues that with so many deaths, if our efforts could accelerate a solution even just a single day, we might save thousands of lives.

It was a furious pace and there wasn't much time for reflection. At one point, however, I noticed similarities to some frantic days in 1974. That wasn't a health crisis, but rather a financial pandemic. Stocks had fallen 50 percent; interest rates doubled; and credit controls had been imposed.

Forty-six years later, I was juggling calls and emails around the world

---

* Johns Hopkins University CSSE COVID-19 Data. The death rate rose and fell in waves. Over the first two years of the pandemic, Hopkins reported an average of more than eight thousand deaths every day.

with doctors, scientists, patients, biotech executives, large employers, vaccine makers, members of Congress, and the media. In 1974, I was directly in the arena with the skills, knowledge and contacts to have an immediate impact on the outcome of the financial crisis. In 2020, however, the crisis called for a different approach. I'm not a doctor or a scientist, not a government health official or pharmaceutical executive. But I had spent decades working to accelerate medical solutions and knew how to deploy human and financial capital.

Fortunately, we had laid the groundwork by building a wide-ranging health network starting at the 2004 *FasterCures* Lake Tahoe Retreat. The network expanded year by year to include relationships in industry, government, academia, the philanthropic and investment communities, and disease-specific organizations.

With this network in place, I held early conversations with Mark Suzman, the head of the Gates Foundation; Richard Hatchett, CEO of the Coalition for Epidemic Preparedness Innovations (CEPI); Eric Schmidt, Google's former chairman; Steve Ballmer, former CEO of Microsoft; Alex Azar, the secretary of Health and Human Services; and other cabinet officers. NIH Director Francis Collins assigned a senior aide to work with us. Unlike the financial crisis of 1974, it was clear to me that government would have to play an essential role in partnership with philanthropies, venture capitalists, and industry. Only government could backstop companies that were being asked to risk expanding manufacturing capacity with no guarantee that the resulting products would work. In this situation, everyone needed to be part of the conversation.

The long days were exhausting, but reports from the front lines of the pandemic—especially the dedication of doctors, nurses, first responders, and others—impelled us to maximum efforts. It was especially heartbreaking to hear of COVID patients dying alone, cut off from loved ones forbidden to give them comfort in their final hours.

FROM INFORMATION TO ACTION

Still, we wanted to reach more people. *What can we do to magnify the impact of our work?* That's when we began using podcasts featuring interviews with global leaders of the COVID response. We sought a wide range of guests chosen carefully for their specific expertise.* One goal was to connect groups whose efforts were complementary. The interviews included physicians, Nobel laureates in science, philanthropists, military leaders, top government officials, major employers, and CEOs of the primary companies developing vaccines and advanced therapeutics. My impatience came through in some of my questions: Why do we need to wait nine months before launching clinical trials of therapies that can save lives? What new initiatives are most likely to change the history of this pandemic? How can we help?

After interacting with and challenging leaders like the NIH director, pharma CEOs and scientists, I saw that the problem wasn't just producing vaccines. The bigger challenge was distributing them and convincing people to take them.

Another issue was the prevalence of distrust in our society. It has many causes including social media, political polarization and international disinformation campaigns. Large percentages of the population don't believe—or don't want to believe—the pronouncements of well-informed authorities. Conspiracy theories put the lives of millions at risk. The podcasts were part of an effort to counter this with useful information.

---

* See www.fastercuresbook.com. After we finished recording the first fifty podcasts, I began branching out to broader topics including food access, financial safety nets, social justice, and the difficult trade-offs policymakers face when trying to slow the spread of a respiratory virus without creating other health, economic or social crises.

Several pharmaceutical and biotechnology competitors began helping each other produce vaccines and therapies: Merck with Johnson & Johnson; Sanofi with GlaxoSmithKline; Pfizer with BioNTech; Eli Lilly with AbCellera; Roche with Regeneron; and others. Some companies opened their patent libraries so others around the world could manufacture products without royalties. CEPI, the Coalition for Epidemic Preparedness Innovation, partnered with individual philanthropists, governments, and private companies.

As we moved from information to action, *FasterCures* launched the COVID-19 Treatment and Vaccine Tracker to increase collaboration, minimize clinical trials duplication, and provide a clearer regulatory pathway for research groups. This tool was adopted by publications around the world including the *Washington Post*, which leveraged our data to drive their graphic visualizations of vaccine development. I suggested to *FasterCures* executive director Esther Krofah that she update the tracker at least once a week. She laughed and told me they were going to update it every day. That was just one of the incredible commitments our employees made throughout the crisis. They worked to minimize funding delays and collaborated with the US Biomedical Advanced Research and Development Authority (BARDA) and several vaccine developers to speed the ramp-up of manufacturing.

RISK AND REWARD

We were also meeting online with dozens of start-ups and small biotech firms to assess who had the most promising products that needed capital. As I later told the *Wall Street Journal*, we've always been a clearinghouse for treatments that showed promise, but which might not make it to market for various commercial or strategic reasons.* At the time, we estimated the pandemic's cost was at least $1 trillion dollars a month, an estimate we later increased. Our goal was to reduce the time needed to discover more effective treatments and vaccines.

Simultaneously, we wanted to work with regulators on finding ways to shorten the clinical trials process. Our message was identical to what we told the FDA about cancer trials in 1995: Accelerate the process by compressing Phase 1 through Phase 3 trials. Would there be risks? Of course. But COVID's toll was already being compared to World War II. And, as General Colin Powell said a quarter century earlier, "In war you take risks based on incomplete information. We send nineteen-year-olds into war zones knowing that no matter what we do, some number greater than zero will lose their lives." We can't tell a desperate COVID patient facing death not to try an experimental drug because it might be dangerous.†

Under the direction of Esther Krofah, *FasterCures* worked closely

---

* Mene Ukueberuwa, "The Weekend Interview with Michael Milken," *Wall Street Journal*, May 1, 2020.

† At the height of the crisis, my mother developed a cough and started to run a fever. At age ninety-eight, she's still sharp, whether playing a hand of bridge, commenting on world affairs, or enjoying an ice cream sundae with chocolate sauce. (Hey, she's ninety-eight—I don't lecture her about nutrition!) Yet, with COVID-19 spreading rapidly and vaccines not yet available, we needed to take extra precautions. "If I have this thing," she said in no uncertain terms, "I'd rather die at home than go to the hospital." Home was the same house she and my father bought more than seventy years ago, the same house where my brother Lowell, my sister Joni and I grew up. As Lori and I, along with Lowell and Joni, were discussing a plan for different scenarios, we learned that she had tested positive for COVID-19. We made sure she had nursing care around the clock to monitor her vital signs and administer antiviral therapies. One night she asked if she was dying. The nurse assured her she was not dying, but had a respiratory infection that would soon get better. We visited her several times a day and she improved over a period of weeks. It was a difficult time as we struggled with whether we'd ever want to override her do-not-resuscitate directive. I'm grateful we didn't have to face that decision. We've since enjoyed more holidays, birthdays, and Mother's Days with Mom.

with the Duke-Margolis Center for Health Policy. They helped develop master protocols to get more people enrolled in COVID-19 clinical trials. They also focused on the special needs of community hospitals and long-term-care facilities to adapt these protocols to their unique situations.

AMAZING COLLABORATION

The global effort to confront the coronavirus crisis wasn't perfect, but it was effective and fast. In December 2020, the FDA gave emergency use authorization to the Pfizer-BioNTech and Moderna vaccines. This was a mere thirty-eight weeks after the first experimental compound was injected into a human volunteer. On one of the early podcasts, David Baltimore said, "There has never been a larger international effort to deal with an infection. That alone makes me optimistic."

Summing up all the efforts by thousands of researchers around the world, former PCF president/CEO Jonathan Simons said, "This is why we all went into medicine—for moments like this where we all come together."

COVID'S LESSONS

The late Armand Hammer used to tell a story, undoubtedly apocryphal, about a business trip to Moscow during the cold war. Looking out of the meeting room window during a negotiation, he saw two men with shovels. The first worker dug a hole in the ground; then his partner filled the hole back in and they moved on to another street. When Dr. Hammer asked what was happening, his host explained that the two men were part of a three-man tree-planting crew; the third man, whose job was to place trees in the holes, was out sick that day.

The story made a humorous point about the inefficiencies of the Soviet system. I gained further insight into that system in the late 1980s when Dr. Hammer and I attended a meeting with General Secretary Mikhail Gorbachev at the Soviet embassy in Washington. Last in the line of Soviet leaders, Mr. Gorbachev and some of his colleagues asked me to explain American corporate finance. He said his nation sought to build a venture capital industry. I told them that VC firms invest in many companies knowing that most will fail, but also knowing that a few big successes can more than pay for the losses on the companies that don't make it. At that point, the Soviet commissar for industry jumped in to say that in his country the failed business executives would never be heard from again. That's when I told them they were not ready for venture capital.

We knew that only a few of the hundreds of projects to develop vaccines for COVID-19 would make it all the way through clinical trials and approval. In fact, the NIH and BARDA achieved their successes against COVID-19 by placing their bets on many promising candidates for new tests, therapies, and vaccines. They acted like venture capitalists; and like VCs, they learned from the failures as well as the successes. The Milken Institute's *FasterCures* staff worked long and hard to keep communication flowing smoothly between private organizations and government regulators.

Other Institute centers fulfilled different roles. Our Center for Financial Markets created programs to shore up small and medium businesses in need of capital. They also helped design food security programs of the Federal Emergency Management Agency as part of FEMA's National Advisory Council. The Milken Institute Center for Public Health collaborated with the Treasury Department and others to create a financial safety net in minority communities designated as "deserts" in terms of access to nutritious food, medical care, and banking services. Our Center for the Future of Aging focused on the most vulnerable seniors. The Center for Strategic Philanthropy coordinated activities of philanthropic foundations and individuals seeking guidance on where their help was most needed.

WHAT WE LEARNED

Historians tell us that plagues and pandemics have often been humanity's feared companions. Each horrific episode delivered useful lessons. Among COVID's lessons:

- Count on the science. The first experiments showing that polio could be transmitted between animals took place in 1908. It took forty-six years before the first approved human vaccine was released in 1954. When the 1918 pandemic hit, scientists knew far less about what they were dealing with. It wasn't until the 1930s that anyone actually saw a virus under a microscope. NIH Director Francis Collins told me that as recently as 2003, it took 149 days before we had even a partial sequence of the SARS-1 virus; for the 2009 swine flu, it took 77 days; SARS-CoV-2 took only 12 days. Each crisis accelerates the science. If we build a better global surveillance system and continue to improve sequencing speeds, we can have almost-instantaneous awareness of another novel coronavirus, an emerging antibiotic-resistant bacterium or a biological terrorist attack.

- Inventing vaccines, therapies, and tests doesn't mean people will use them. The rate of polio vaccinations in America skyrocketed after Elvis Presley bared his arm for a polio shot on national television in 1956. There is no Elvis today—only millions of often-misinformed people espousing various theories on social media. Much of the population refuses COVID testing even though it's easy, fast, and free. This is more than frustrating—it's deadly. In fact, more people have died from COVID *after* vaccines became widely available than before. That's not because the vaccines are ineffective. It's just that people too often believe false information. It does no good to lecture people. Lacking a reincarnation of Elvis, we just have to continue providing factual education.

+ <u>Our systems are resilient.</u> No matter how severe the crisis, many services we rely on continued to work well. The internet, financial markets, electric grids, water supply, gas pipelines, long-haul trucking, mail delivery—the infrastructure of everyday life—mostly held up fine.

+ <u>The response could have been faster.</u> A virus spreads quickly. We should have had a better early warning system and a better plan in place. America wasn't ready.

+ <u>Inequities persist.</u> No one is surprised that the most vulnerable groups in our population suffered the most. We can do much more to address disparities based on race, gender, ethnicity and age.

+ <u>Public health matters.</u> We have traditionally devoted more than 85 percent of healthcare dollars to caring for patients and less than 15 percent to prevention and research. Public health measures to contain COVID—including such basic advice as hand washing and mask wearing—saved lives early in the pandemic and contributed to a decline in cases of seasonal influenza.

+ <u>The definition of "essential workers" expanded.</u> We used to think of nurses, doctors, and first responders—police, firefighters, EMTs—as the essential workers most deserving of our appreciation. We now also recognize our growing dependence on many others such as grocery store clerks and delivery truck drivers.

+ <u>Big pharma was effective.</u> The day-and-night dedication of pharmaceutical and biotechnology company employees produced vaccines and therapeutics in an unbelievably short time. That saved tens of millions of lives.

+ Distribution planning was disappointing. While vaccine development was miraculous, we should have been planning distribution logistics much earlier. After a lot of confusion, some observers concluded the most effective system would have been simply to allocate vaccines by age. Whether or not that's the right process, what's clear is that hundreds of US state and local agencies went in every direction and far too many consumers didn't know where to turn.

+ Build manufacturing capacity before it's needed. In normal circumstances, pharmaceutical companies can't take the risk of investing in large-scale production of medicines before clinical trials are complete and the FDA approves. The Operation Warp Speed team understood that many people could die while waiting for a vaccine. Therefore, BARDA contracted with industry for pre-approval manufacturing. In other words, they paid in advance for products that might have to be discarded if they weren't approved. It wasn't a perfect process, but it saved many lives. Before the next crisis, we should be building new manufacturing facilities and warehousing strategic supplies.

+ Don't put all the eggs in one basket. Winning the war against a pandemic means fighting battles on several fronts: testing, vaccine development, public health strategies, and accelerated R&D on new treatments. Even while the Milken Institute COVID-19 Treatment and Vaccine Tracker eventually identified some 269 vaccine-development programs, another 332 treatments were moving through the pipeline toward approval. These included monoclonal antibodies, antivirals, immune modulators, cell-based therapies, mechanical devices, RNA-based treatments, and repurposed compounds.

+ A better flu vaccine may be coming. During the twentieth century, development of antibiotics controlled most bacterial infections. Now we're closing in on solutions to major viral diseases including a universal flu vaccine. The global effort to combat COVID-19 accelerated this broader work. Several manufacturers are working on easier-to-administer vaccine formulations.

With the benefit of hindsight, it's clear we could have done many things differently. When the nation focused on vaccine development in 2020, we should have had a broader focus on areas like distribution. In some cases, well-meaning efforts to protect people did more damage than the virus itself. We should analyze the pros and cons of specific actions like lockdowns and school closings so we're better informed for the next crisis.

We're still learning in a number of areas—how, for example, to confront the long-term mental health needs of society in a "new normal." But considering the all-encompassing global disruption that COVID-19 caused, it might have been far worse.

PREPARING FOR THE NEXT CRISIS

The COVID-19 pandemic was a world war—a war of science against disease. Its decline is not the end of health crises. Epidemiologists agree that the SARS-CoV-2 virus and its variants are unlikely to disappear completely. They also warn that an even-deadlier pathogen might launch the next pandemic. If any good is to come from the recent tragedy, surely it must be that the world will be better prepared next time. While nearly everyone agrees about readiness in principle, agreement could vanish quickly if nations regress into political squabbles over spending and control.

Preparation for the next crisis should begin with an understanding that pandemics don't arise in a vacuum. They spread on the winds of what tropical disease specialist Peter Hotez calls "wider global currents." These include political instability, climate change, social media misinformation and anti-science crusades.

CHEAP INSURANCE

"COVID-19 caught the world by surprise," says *FasterCures* Executive Director Esther Krofah. "It shouldn't have." To the extent that it exists, the current system for detecting pandemics by governments and private organizations is woefully fragmented and slow. Instead of waiting for local disease outbreaks, then noting them manually, then notifying the World Health Organization, we need a proactive, automated system. This could compress months of delay into hours and save untold numbers of lives.

FasterCures is working to help implement a better system, but the greater challenge will be securing buy-in on who controls it and who pays for it. Economists and epidemiologists will tell you the world could save millions of lives and trillions of dollars by spending a few billions of dollars in the short term. We haven't done that adequately in the past because public health and research funding has always suffered from boom-and-bust cycles.

We spend less than a billion dollars a year on pandemic preparedness. I believe it will take many times that amount to create an effective shield. It's still a small number next to the cost of COVID-19—estimated by the International Monetary Fund at more than $30 *trillion*. Think of it as cheap insurance.

ADDRESSING INEQUALITY

The pandemic caused millions of businesses to fail; it also exposed inadequate support for minority-owned banks and tremendous disparities in the healthcare system. Mellody Hobson, co-CEO of Ariel Investments and chairwoman of Starbucks, is a highly successful African American business executive. She pointed out on one of my podcasts that the finances of Black and brown women—employees and business owners alike—were especially hard hit. We need to address these societal issues as urgently as we attack the disease itself.

Other forms of "collateral damage" from the pandemic are extremely serious, if not as widely noted. For example, the National Cancer Institute has projected 4,500 excess deaths from colon cancer by 2030 because of delayed diagnoses and treatment. The Alzheimer's Association says deaths from that disease were 16 percent higher than expected in 2020. During the pandemic's first wave, panicked patients who feared infection risks in doctors' offices and hospitals delayed treatment for chronic conditions. Many even avoided emergency treatment for life-threatening episodes. The hospital administrators I spoke to reported reductions as high as 40 percent in reported cancer, heart attacks, and strokes.[*]

Over the long term, deaths will be higher because of clinical trials that were disrupted, suspended, delayed or canceled. Some laboratories had to close because scientists were pulled away to work on COVID.

Delays in age-dependent childhood immunizations put millions at risk worldwide. We were close to finally stamping out polio in the few countries where it persists. Now that goal is in the future as the incidence of polio rises. This backsliding on immunizations is one of

---

[*] Patients who have failed treatments elsewhere often turn to the NCI Hospital for its leading-edge treatments. There's always a long waiting list for its limited number of beds. Yet in the weeks after the crisis began, the NCI's Steve Rosenberg told me that many of its hallways were virtually deserted. During that same period, John Mazziota, CEO of UCLA Health, said his always-crowded emergency room was all but empty. Nobel laureate Jim Allison commented that research ground to a halt.

COVID's most tragic consequences. Lockdowns in the poorest developing countries also halted what had been encouraging progress against tuberculosis, measles, dengue and malaria.

So-called deaths of despair were a persistent problem before COVID. Suicides increased during the pandemic and fatal drug overdoses rose sharply. Spousal and child abuse, often unreported, are believed to have followed a tragically upward trend.

EARLY WARNING

We've learned from this pandemic and can be much better prepared if we're careful not to slip back to the old ways. We have new technology for sequencing the genomes of virus samples quickly and inexpensively. We didn't sequence enough COVID-19 samples early in the pandemic and that lack of genomic surveillance limited the ability to recognize mutations. "Without that data," says *FasterCures's* Esther Krofah, "we're flying blind." An effective national program using gene-mapping technology will cost a few billion dollars. Let's invest in it now so our scientific infrastructure is prepared to pounce on any new pathogen next time.

One overriding message of this pandemic is that none of us is safe unless all of us are safe. Whether they're in Kenya or Kentucky, Brazil or Boston, Vietnam or Vermont, people move around. Any new virus could turn into a new global emergency. Former NIH Director Elias Zerhouni says, "You can't close your borders and say, 'Okay, we're going to be safe.'" He believes existing international groups—WHO, GAVI, CEPI, and others—can play important roles.

Dr. Scott Gottlieb, my colleague on the *FasterCures* board and a former FDA commissioner, has an interesting perspective on this issue. He says that coordination of public health agencies across borders, though helpful, isn't enough.

> To promptly collect this kind of information, we can't rely only on public health agencies and their tools of international collaboration in known hot spots. Our government has the capacity to gather epidemiological facts even when other nations don't want to share them. Deploying intelligence agencies to monitor outbreaks would advance our public health goals and help guard against adversaries who would try to exploit the chaos brought on by a health crisis.[*]

Scott suggests the Defense Department "reprogram its biodefense resources" to focus on combating viruses, which are "far more accessible than enriched uranium and easier to engineer, but still capable of unleashing mass destruction."

DOUBLE DOWN ON WHAT WORKS

In addition to creating a more effective warning system, we must continue to expand support for the next generation of researchers, build vaccine manufacturing capacity *before* it's needed, and involve patients more completely in R&D. These efforts cannot be limited to the wealthy developed nations. Because pandemics are by definition global, we need competent vaccine developers and manufacturers throughout the world. Moving forward, we must do better.

Unfortunately, the lessons of pandemics tend to fade from memory. Now is the time to double down on what has worked well. Just

---

* Scott Gottlieb, "Intelligence Agencies Can Help Stop Future Pandemics," *Washington Post*, September 17, 2001.

as America created NASA and DARPA in response to Sputnik, the nation needs a permanent force to confront emerging health threats. COVID-19 is our new Sputnik moment. Let us use it to recommit to bioscience progress and preparedness on behalf of all the world's people.

TWENTY-ONE

Data and Technology

———

Jennifer Doudna's path to scientific prominence began in Hilo on the Big Island of Hawaii, far from the centers of technology development. She grew up at a time when few girls "did science." But she loved detective stories, found the variety of nature awesome, and had an insatiable desire to figure out how living things work. That desire—combined with her brilliant mind and dedication to hard work—has put her at the center of the greatest revolution in human history: the cracking of life's genetic code. We now have the power, should we choose to use it, to alter evolution.

When Jennifer first joined us at the Milken Institute Global Conference a decade ago, she was known within the scientific community as an expert on RNA, a subject overshadowed by media coverage of its DNA cousin. I interviewed her and recognized the same curiosity that has always driven me to devour statistics. It was the first time we heard the term CRISPR and not the last time we considered its ethical implications.* Even then, Jennifer appreciated the great need for social responsibility in developing a powerful gene-editing technology with the potential to change humanity.

Only a few years later, a rogue Chinese scientist announced the birth of three babies produced from human embryos whose genes had been altered for resistance to the HIV virus. The implication that parents might someday be able to choose their children's genetic characteristics—height, eye color, athletic ability, or intelligence—has raised profound concerns, as it should. Yet the same technology has the potential to reduce immense human suffering from gene-linked diseases including Alzheimer's and cancer.

JUST THE BEGINNING

CRISPR, to give an oversimplified explanation of a complex technology, is a way to edit some of the letters in a genome. That could make plants more nutritious and drought-resistant, take the allergens out of peanuts, cure AIDS, wipe out malaria-transmitting mosquitoes, or inactivate the COVID-19 virus. The possibilities are endless.

Despite obvious risks, CRISPR is so significant that it earned the 2020 Nobel Prize in Chemistry for Dr. Doudna at Berkeley, and her colleague, Emmanuelle Charpentier, a French scientist. They showed that a characteristic of bacterial immune systems could be used to make precise cuts in any sequence of DNA letters. It is, says Doudna, "literally a way that bacteria fight viral infection."

---

* An internet search will yield thousands of articles about CRISPR (clustered regularly interspaced short palindromic repeats), many of which are highly technical. Here's a relatively nontechnical article that gives a good overview: https://www.vox.com/2018/7/23/17594864/crispr-cas9-gene-editing. Also, see Walter Isaacson's book, *The Code Breaker: Jennifer Doudna, Gene Editing, and the Future of the Human Race*, Simon & Schuster, 2021.

A few weeks before the Nobel Prize announcement, Jennifer joined me on one of my podcasts and explained that the process of editing a single gene is relatively straightforward. It gets far more complex when it comes to treating human diseases. That's because many different genes may be involved and medical researchers don't yet fully understand the endless ways they interact. For example, nearly 300 genes have been identified as contributors to cancer. A few hereditary conditions, however, arise from a single defective gene. One of them is sickle cell disease. Jennifer talked about the first patient to receive a CRISPR gene-editing treatment:

> I'm really excited that on sickle cell disease, the technology has already been shown to work. Some people may have seen the announcements about Victoria Gray who received a CRISPR treatment. She is now more than a year out and is effectively cured, which is just extraordinary. It's incredibly inspiring to see her life changed in such a positive way.
>
> Another great example is treating a neurodegenerative condition such as Parkinson's or Huntington's disease, and maybe at some point even things like ALS or Alzheimer's disease. This is not going to happen overnight. This is not going to happen even in the next couple of years. But I think that many of us working in the field can see the opportunities.

Later in our talk, Jennifer and I discussed COVID-19 and cancer. While she was cautious about speculating on cures, she was sure that further development of the technique will eventually allow it to be applied to "anything that has a unique sequence of DNA or RNA."*

---

* In June 2021, Jennifer Doudna announced another milestone in the potential application of CRISPR technology—the direct editing of DNA in humans after systemic delivery of a therapeutic agent. Previously, cells had to be removed from the body before editing.

That process has moved quickly since our 2021 conversation: Experimental drugs that use an updated CRISPR technology called base editing are now in clinical trials to test whether they can permanently lower cholesterol and restore insulin production to type 1 diabetes patients.

It may be years before this technology is widely available to patients. In its current stage of development, I'm reminded of Winston Churchill's comment following an early British victory in World War II: "This is not the end. It is not even the beginning of the end. But it is, perhaps, the end of the beginning." CRISPR is an exciting beginning in the search for faster cures.

SPEED, COST, STORAGE, AND ACCESS

The common characteristic of all new technologies like CRISPR is their reliance on the collection and processing of data. If the biological sciences are to our time what physics was to the last century, it is largely because the code of life—the four base components of DNA—can be processed in the same way that the binary code of zeros and ones underlies everything we do in our electronic devices.

In the 1967 movie *The Graduate*, Dustin Hoffman stars as a twenty-one-year-old who's unsure about his career path. An older man pulls him aside and says, "I just want to say one word to you. Just one word. Are you listening? Plastics! There's a great future in plastics." If a new version of the Academy Award–winning comedy were being made today, that line would have to be updated. The one word would probably be "bioscience."

The driving force behind the impact of bioscience on our lives and health is the astounding advance of our ability to produce, manipulate, store, retrieve, and transmit data. Plummeting processing costs, increased transfer speeds, virtually unlimited electronic storage capacity, instant communication, and universal access to mobile devices have been consistent themes in hundreds of my speeches over the past thirty years.

When I was a child, the most valuable companies were in smoke-stack industries like steel and automobile manufacturing. Today, the market leaders are firms like Apple, Microsoft, Amazon and Alphabet—all built on data. Each has benefited from the same speed, cost and storage trends that drive medical progress.

As a result, bioscience investigators now have the tools to prevent immense suffering by testing patients' DNA for variations that link to specific diseases. Their ability to find these variations increased rapidly over the years. In 1987, a *New York Times* article reported:

> *Only about 500 human genes (less than one percent of the total) have been decoded. Scientists are slogging through the human genome like a third-grader reading Kierkegaard. Even a steady rise in the rate of sequencing would leave the job unfinished until the 22nd century.*

Six years after that discouraging analysis, I met Dr. Jonathan Simons at Johns Hopkins. He reported that he could read five hundred letters of the human genome every day. At that rate, it would have taken 167,000 years to process a full genome.

DEVOTION TO SCIENCE

Fortunately, that's when Dr. Francis Collins* assumed leadership of the Human Genome Project at the National Center for Human

---

* Francis Collins and I first met at his induction into the American Academy of Achievement in 1993. I'd been inducted into the Academy in 1985. The 1993 event was in Las

Genome Research in the NIH. Within a decade, Francis and his colleagues announced the first working draft of the entire human genome, an effort that cost nearly $3 billion and involved a consortium of 2,400 scientists in six countries. It was a scientific *tour de force* comparable to the splitting of the atom or the moon landing.

The Genome Project set out first to determine the exact order of the three billion base pairs ("letters") on the twenty-three pairs of chromosomes in all our cell nuclei; then to create physical and genetic maps of the genome in humans and other organisms. In June 2000, the consortium completed the rough draft of the genome sequence. Less than three years later, a more complete version was made public. The final "truly complete map" of the genome—the first gapless sequence—was announced in 2022. It should accelerate the search for cures to several more genetic diseases in areas like aging, the brain, cancer, and heart disease. As Nobel laureate David Baltimore wrote in *Nature*, "The human genome holds an extraordinary trove of information about human development, physiology, medicine, and evolution." Virtually all the recent advances in biotechnology have built on this structure. It is, according to an article on the NIH website, "similar to having all the pages of a manual needed to make the human body."

Such momentous achievements would have been hard to predict given Francis's humble beginnings. He grew up on a farm in Virginia's Shenandoah Valley, where his boyhood home had no indoor bathroom. He loved to read and developed a passion for chemistry. He was studying for a PhD in physical chemistry at Yale when he

---

Vegas at the Mirage Hotel, a project my company had financed. Francis had just begun his work as Director of the National Human Genome Research Institute where he would lead the historic effort to decipher the code of life. Twenty-eight years later, in December 2021, I delivered a talk congratulating Francis on his completion of a twelve-year tenure as head of the National Institutes of Health. He is the only presidentially appointed NIH Director ever to have served under three presidents.

took a molecular biology course that opened his eyes to the potential of DNA, especially in medicine.

That early fascination evolved into a career of relentless gene hunting. Francis led teams credited with discovering the genes responsible for cystic fibrosis, Huntington's disease, neurofibromatosis, multiple endocrine neoplasia type 1, and the M4 type of adult acute leukemia. He and his team also identified the genetic basis of Hutchinson-Gilford progeria syndrome, a tragic condition that causes premature aging. "Besides opening the door to possible treatment strategies for progeria," he says, "the discovery may provide insights into the process of normal human aging."

Francis was looking forward to continuing this work when he stepped down from his executive role as NIH director and returned to his laboratory. But within months, President Biden asked him to take on the temporary role of science advisor to the president and cochair of the President's Council of Advisors on Science and Technology.

SEQUENCING AND ARTIFICIAL INTELLIGENCE

The cost of whole-genome sequencing continues to fall dramatically. As this is written, genome sequencing for as low as $100 is within sight. At that level, it could be practical to incorporate it into a routine physical exam.

Another result of cheaper sequencing is the growth of artificial intelligence applications. AI has great promise, but also significant limitations. Commenting on the current state of AI technology at the 2022 Milken Institute Global Conference, former Google chairman Eric Schmidt noted that we're happy to have it forecast the weather, but we're not ready to have it fly passenger airplanes.

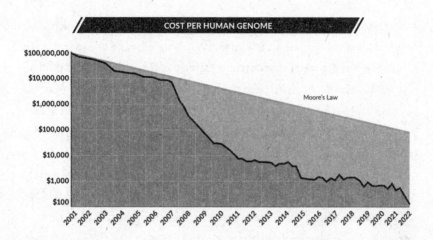

Sources: Illumina, Inc. and genome.gov.

One thing AI does very well is to extract useful information from enormous amounts of raw data. It can, for example, rapidly survey millions of symptoms, cases, and articles to produce a likely diagnosis. Dr. David Feinberg, currently the head of Cerner, a division of Oracle Corporation, was one of the first leaders of a major medical center to implement this capability. When David was CEO of Geisinger Health System in Pennsylvania, he installed the first AI programs to review all CAT scans and MRIs. Before the doctors even saw these scans, the computer had prioritized them and suggested diagnoses.

AI is very also useful in certain other areas—as a robotic teacher, for example, it is infinitely patient in assisting students with dyslexia or autism. It can handle many discrete tasks such as image and pattern recognition: Is that mole on your arm benign or potentially malignant? Is the shadow on your lung X-ray serious or not? Do subtle changes in your speech signify early Alzheimer's? Where AI falls short today is in its understanding of a complex set of signs and symptoms in an individual patient from a particular social setting interacting face-to-face with an experienced clinician. The best doctors see the entire patient, not just the test numbers. AI is great with numbers, but currently lacks the creativity of a highly trained doctor.

Dr. Richard Merkin recognized the power of AI to process numbers when he created the $3 million Heritage Health Prize Competition. Dick is the founder and CEO of the Heritage Group, the largest, physician-owned and-operated integrated health delivery system in America. His unique prize challenge asked a deceptively simple question: Is it possible to predict with great accuracy who in a large population of patients is most likely to be hospitalized in the next year? The competition attracted 39,000 entries from forty-one countries. The resulting algorithms are helping providers and insurance companies deliver interventions that keep people healthier. I've long admired Dick's creativity and invited him to join us as one of the original founders of *FasterCures*.

One of the most significant AI breakthroughs is proteomics, which greatly extends the genomic revolution's impact. Nobel laureate Frances Arnold, a Caltech professor, offers a dramatic explanation of the practical benefits. Before the genome project, she said, there was no way to select for specific properties of a protein that might be hundreds of amino acids long. It reminded her of the story "The Library of Babel" by Jorge Luis Borges. The order and content of the library's books was completely random, which made it impossible to find even one coherent sentence. The massive computing power of today's processors solves this problem with profound implications in such areas as pharmacology, agriculture, and renewable energy.

Using proteomics, scientists have recently figured out solutions to the "protein folding problem." Proteins are molecules, made up of strings of amino acids, that control every function (and every dysfunction) of the human body. Their three-dimensional structure is basically determined by the sequence of twenty different amino acids, which cause them to fold and loop around in shapes so complex and limitless that they've been virtually impossible to describe in mathematical terms, much less predict how different shapes affect the health of the entire body.

It's a riddle that biologists and biophysicists have tried to solve for sixty years. The British laboratory DeepMind, which is owned by Google's parent, Alphabet, solved the problem using a neural network technology called AlphaFold, a form of AI. For nearly all of the human body's hundred-million-plus protein structures, DeepMind can predict their shape with considerable accuracy based on the amino-acid sequence. It's enormously important because knowing what shape a protein will fold into is a major step in finding another molecule—a drug or vaccine—that will lock onto that shape. This may transform biomedicine. "It's an extraordinary advance," says Eric Schmidt. "It allows new drugs to be designed that would have been beyond the capacity of humans to create. That's the beginning of general intelligence in machines."

Illumina, Inc., of San Diego, is a leading driver of these trends. They've helped bring down the costs of analyzing gene variations by a factor of more than a million in two decades. Illumina is led by Ethiopian-born Francis deSouza, who came to America at the age of sixteen to attend MIT. When I spoke to him recently, Francis pointed out the potential of genome sequencing:

"We believe that ninety-five percent of all human diseases have a genetic component; yet today we understand only fifteen percent. We're working to understand which patients are most vulnerable based on their genome and protect them. Prenatal testing is one such area since five percent of newborns have some kind of genetic disease. If a baby's genome is sequenced at birth, you can get a diagnosis in about half the cases. That can save years of suffering for the child as well as anguish and expense for parents."

I asked Francis about storing data on strands of DNA, instead of in memory chips. This incredibly dense storage medium could theoretically hold all the world's knowledge in a shoebox. He agreed that DNA has been optimized by nature to be the best medium and "it's only a matter of time" until we use it to store data. That holds the promise of even faster speeds and lower costs in accessing data.

TECHNOLOGY AND OUR HEALTH

Hundreds of technological advances are accelerating progress in every corner of medicine. Here are a dozen of them:

1. Physicians can target cancers more precisely with the right drugs in the right amounts at the right time with fewer side effects because they can now sequence the tumor itself. They no longer have to guess about the genetic makeup based on its location in the body. This often allows cancer patients to replace chemotherapy with less toxic, more effective treatments. New drugs targeting a specific mutation (called KRAS) common to many cancers help patients survive longer, compared to chemotherapy, before their tumors get worse.

2. Researchers have already discovered genes associated with more than five thousand rare diseases and can see patterns of gene expression in individual cells.

3. Scientific understanding of the immune system, blood components, and the microbiome has grown by orders of magnitude over twenty years. Our increased ability to sequence gut microbes is unlocking the microbiome's secrets in ways that can personalize nutrition to fight disease more effectively.

4. After the COVID lockdown in 2020, telemedicine took off. Many doctors had more online encounters with patients in a

day than in all of 2019.* We will never go back to the old model of driving to a doctor's office for every medical reason.

5. Two decades ago, minimally invasive surgery began to replace many types of traditional operations. Now we're starting to see new types of <u>non</u>invasive surgery, such as focused ultrasound, for hundreds of procedures.

6. "Smart bomb" drugs combine potent toxins with antibodies that target only specific types of cancer cells. Researchers at Stanford University have created miniature robots that may one day crawl through our bodies releasing drugs at specific locations. With a similar technology, Perdue University neurosurgeons are testing "microbots" to remove blood from the brain after a stroke.

7. As microbes mutate and become resistant to existing antibiotics, rapid sequencing of infectious organisms is helping researchers trying to stay a step ahead of these dangerous new bugs. That sequencing has also increased the ability of epidemiologists to predict the course of pandemics more accurately.

8. Natural language processing now allows doctors to interrogate databases without entering complex formulas. For example, they can ask, "What percentage of patients with condition X also have condition Y?"

9. The lead time for vaccine development is getting shorter. What used to take years can be completed in days. The rapid development of COVID-19 vaccines showed that as soon as a data set is complete, it can be uploaded to the internet, where it's available to the world's scientific community.

---

* Some primary care physicians are concerned about losing touch, literally, with their patients; but various surveys have shown that more than four out of five patients say these telehealth visits are as good as or better than an in-person appointment. They are part of what former Google CEO Eric Schmidt called "tele-everything" on one of my podcasts. "Let's take advantage of the digital infrastructure," he said, "and use it for everyday things."

10. The precision of medical imaging now shows anatomical features thousands of times smaller than just a decade ago. Among many applications, this technology can see tiny tumors that traditional scans would miss. Just as important, these images can be read anywhere in the world.

11. By harnessing artificial intelligence, machine learning, and massive computational power, scientists can now design and synthesize drugs from scratch inside a laboratory computer rather than testing thousands of molecules against biological targets. Instead of using test tubes, buffers, and pipettes, scientists study the target structures on a computer screen and test them, digitally, against a library of fifty billion chemical compounds, each a potential medication. Only then do they need to work in a wet lab to validate a particular chemical's theoretical efficacy. This is good news for mice because experiments are computer simulations in silico—no mice need be sacrificed.

12. At some future time, doctors may be able to implant "neural prosthetics" that allow a paralyzed person to create documents on a computer screen simply by thinking about the letters or words. But the future is already here for wearable devices with a wide range of medical applications. Close to 100 million people have wrist sensors that detect such signals as their heart rates. As the physician and entrepreneur Peter Diamandis points out, this allows healthcare to move out of the doctor's office and hospital to our own bodies. He foresees the routine implantation of radio-frequency chips under the skin to measure dozens of blood parameters and other signs of disease. With the patient's permission, artificial intelligence programs will analyze the data in search of relevant patterns. As data from millions of devices are consolidated and correlated with disease patterns, the programs will become smarter and more predictive. Asked about the cost of such monitoring, Peter replies, "What's the cost of treating stage IV cancer compared to catching it at stage I?" Wearable

devices could be particularly helpful in dealing with high blood pressure, which causes more deaths and disability than any underlying condition. Seventy percent of patients do not have their hypertension under control. Because it's difficult to get an accurate baseline reading in a doctor's office, we need a system of twenty-four-hour ambulatory measurement. The commercial appeal of such a wearable monitor is clear and should provide the incentive for industry development.

This trend toward healthcare centered on people rather than buildings reminds me of my first encounter with Craig McCaw, a visionary businessman who saw a future that many large corporations missed. In the late 1970s, AT&T decided not to pursue the mobile telephone business when a consulting firm estimated there would be a *total* long-term demand of only one million phones. Craig, who with his brothers founded McCaw Cellular Communications, told me, "The consultants mistakenly equated a telephone number to a physical location." But with the mobile cellular networks he was developing, a number would designate a person, not a place. I helped finance the growth of Craig's business and in 1994, he and his brothers sold McCaw Cellular to AT&T for $11.5 billion. The company was renamed AT&T Wireless. By the late 1990s, sales of cell phones exceeded one million *per day.*

The result of these trends, says physician-entrepreneur Arie Belldegrun, is that we're living at a time of life science revolution: "We've now cloned the entire human genome, and every one of those genes is a target for human drugs." Arie notes that twenty years ago, the idea of putting a live cell in a human, directing it to travel to a specific location and do a specific task would have been considered science fiction. Today it's reality and hundreds of companies are working on cell therapy applications.

IT'S ALL IN YOUR BLOOD

My belief in the importance of data goes way back to my childhood collection of World Almanacs. It was always useful to have more facts. In the 1970s, my department acquired what was then the world's most powerful business computer to crunch oceans of data produced on the trading floor.*

It can even be worthwhile to collect more information than you know how to process. Eventually, the technology will catch up. In the 1980s, processing power was increasing exponentially, thanks to Moore's law, and the cost of data storage was dropping even more rapidly. At a 1985 Milken Family Foundation conference, I proposed the idea of storing blood samples in hopes of extracting data from them in the decades to come. Within a decade, it was possible to store and examine millions more samples for what it used to cost us to test and store a few hundred. And today, for the same price, it's billions of samples. Now, a doctor anywhere in the world can analyze a patient's blood thoroughly and inexpensively.

THE NEW MEDICAL EDUCATION

Since genome sequencing can be done so rapidly, physicians are increasingly becoming bioengineers.† Many young doctors have de-

---

* Our IBM model 370–168 was a behemoth that proudly offered eight megabytes of integrated monolithic processor storage at a cost of approximately $1 million per megabyte. That's about 472 million times as expensive per megabyte as the largest capacity Apple iPhone 14 Pro. With 64,000 times as much storage, the phone's cost per megabyte is $0.00212. With access to the cloud, storage is virtually unlimited.

† Medical students finally have access to the types of data sets in bioengineering that are

grees in fields like engineering and data management in addition to medical degrees. They understand the use of large data sets to solve medical problems. The most important impact of this trend is on collaborative research. No longer can a single medical scientist take a discovery from bench to bedside. Science is now a team activity. This is how Dr. Kenneth Pienta puts it:*

Studying medicine in the 1980s was all about memorization. Today, it's who can best gather information from multiple sources and process it. With far more papers being published, it's about who can devise the best search terms. A decade ago in my lab, a multidisciplinary team might involve a medical oncologist, a urologist and a radiation oncologist. Now we'd add to those a cancer biologist, a physicist, an evolutionary ecologist, a bio-physicist, a game theory scientist, a geo-biologist, and an evolutionary dynamics expert; and they'd come from multiple countries.

Ken explains that evolutionary dynamics is the study of how biological organisms evolve according to mathematical principles. And game theory? Evolutionary game theorists apply the applications of game theory to the evolution of biological species—a way of modeling Darwinian competition. (Who knew that cancer cells have to exchange resources with each other and compete to become a successful tumor?) Few doctors-to-be ever studied these disciplines a

---

analogous to the files finance majors took for granted as far back as the 1960s—the computerized CRSP tapes of stock prices that I used as a student at Berkeley.

* Ken Pienta has been at the forefront of cancer research since he first presented the results of his work as a young researcher at our Scientific Retreats more than a quarter century ago. Today, he is the Donald S. Coffey professor of urology and professor of oncology and pharmacology and molecular sciences at the Johns Hopkins University School of Medicine. He is also the director of research at the Brady Urological Institute.

generation ago. Today, biomedical engineering is one of the most important pre-med undergraduate majors.

One key to faster cures is convincing more of those students—young people who could become the next Jennifer Doudna or Francis Collins—to devote their lives to science.

TWENTY-TWO

Our Healthier Future

——————

An MRI technician offered Clark Judge a choice of music before sliding him into the scanning machine's doughnut hole. Clark looked up from the gurney and smiled. "How about the Beatles' *Sergeant Pepper* album?" Soon, the combination of the Fab Four's classic songs and a mild sedative were all Clark needed to actually enjoy final preparations for the next day's brain surgery. Yes, brain surgery—an outpatient procedure using sound waves that involved no anesthesia, cutting, drilling, blood loss, stitches, scarring, infection risk or nights in the hospital. The costs, covered by insurance, were far lower than what traditional open surgery would involve.

Clark is an opinion journalist and founder/CEO of the White House Writers Group, a strategic communications and public affairs firm. Ever since his days as a speechwriter and special assistant to President Reagan, he's been known as one of Washington's most gifted writers. When interviewing a source for an article or speech,

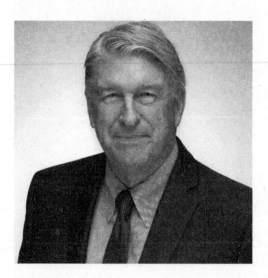

he used to take notes by hand, at least until his smooth penmanship began to deteriorate into an unintelligible scrawl. It was embarrassing and frustrating.

The first doctor Clark consulted diagnosed essential tremor, a progressive neurological disease that often affects control of the hands. It is believed to be caused by misfiring brain neurons. Propranolol, a beta-blocker drug, can help, but is only marginally effective for most patients. Another option is deep brain stimulation, a major surgical procedure that involves drilling holes in the skull and inserting electrodes that are wired under the skin to a neurostimulator device implanted in the chest. Clark didn't want any part of that operation with its long list of risks and its restrictions on his active lifestyle. When a friend said, "You've got to get that fixed," he reached out to me. After we discussed his tremor, I suggested he contact Dr. Neal Kassell, founder of the Focused Ultrasound Foundation, who might offer a solution.

On a chilly January day in 2022, Clark and his wife Margo drove from Washington to a hotel near the University of Maryland Medical Center in Baltimore. The next morning, his scalp was shaved and he was fitted with a metal helmet to make sure his head didn't move during the procedure. His surgeon, Dr. Howard Eisenberg, chair of Maryland's neurosurgery department, sat at a console in an adjacent room. Clark recalls the experience:

> *"I closed my eyes, they slid me in, and I had a good time. Dr. Eisenberg watched real-time images of my brain and directed pulses of focused ultrasound to a very precise spot. It was painless and really quite interesting. Before I knew it, we were done."*

Later that day, Clark met Margo for lunch and they returned to their hotel. "That evening," says Clark, "I asked for a yellow legal pad and a pen. For the first time in more than a decade, effortlessly, fluidly, I signed my name."

NEW TREATMENT OPTIONS

Focused ultrasound is now an approved treatment for essential tremor, as it is for more than sixty other medical indications.* You might remember using focused energy as a kid to burn a hole in a leaf by concentrating beams of sunlight with a magnifying glass. A far-more-sophisticated application of this basic idea concentrates sound waves from multiple directions to pinpoint errant cells that can be zapped without damaging surrounding healthy tissue.

Ultrasonic therapy can successfully treat conditions as diverse as

---

* Focused ultrasound can be very effective for properly selected essential tremor patients. However, neurologists caution that since it makes permanent changes in the brain, it should be recommended only after conservative and reversible treatments have been tried.

uterine fibroids, Parkinson's disease, glaucoma, heart valve calcifications, thyroid cancer, epilepsy, irritable bowel syndrome, and dozens of others. Because it safely crosses the blood-brain barrier, this technology provides new options for treating conditions in the brain.

Other ways science is improving your prospects for a healthier future can be grouped into several broad categories:

- Conditions that have already produced symptoms, especially those affecting the brain and the microbiome.

- Early detection of processes that have not yet produced symptoms including cancer and cardiovascular diseases.

- Progress on slowing the aging process, including restoration or replacement of diseased organs.

- Other advanced technologies for the future.

- What you can do to improve population health . . . and your own.

THE BRAIN AND THE MICROBIOME

The 86 billion neurons and trillions of connections in the human brain are just beginning to yield their secrets. Advanced imaging technologies are allowing investigators to see the brain's circuits for the first time. There's reason for increased hope of progress against all neurodegenerative diseases. Among other benefits, this could forestall the massive suffering and potential economic catastrophe of Alzheimer's disease. Alzheimer's research has been frustrating and slow, but hope is rising that the use of artificial intelligence by laboratory scientists may speed development of more effective drugs.

Meanwhile, the Milken Institute's Center for the Future of Aging has launched the Alliance to Improve Dementia Care. The Alliance seeks to transform the complex health and long-term care systems that people with dementia must navigate.* In other brain-related initiatives, the Institute partnered with the Sergey Brin Family Foundation to design and incubate a global basic science research initiative for Parkinson's disease.

We've also joined the family philanthropies of Sergey Brin, David and Jan Baszucki, and Kent and Liz Dauten, who have collectively committed $150 million to launch BD^2 ("Breakthrough Discoveries for Thriving with Bipolar Disorder"), a program managed by our Center for Strategic Philanthropy. BD^2 will research genetic markers for bipolar disorder with the goal of finding more effective treatments.

Achieving a healthier future will also require major efforts to address the collateral damage of mental health issues. The Milken Institute Center for Public Health calls these issues a shadow crisis. We've created programs to deal with the obesity and drug abuse epidemics that contribute to the crisis and we are spotlighting potential solutions at the Future of Health and other Institute events.

The brain is not the only organ that controls or affects processes elsewhere in the body. Traditional Indian medicine has long considered our guts the "second brain" because of the interactions between the brain and our microbiomes. In recent years, scientists have increased their knowledge of the trillions of bacteria, viruses, fungi, and other microbes that inhabit the digestive tract.† Importantly, the

---

* In late 2022, the Milken Institute released an updated report, "Projected Prevalence and Cost of Dementia." It estimated that treatment expenditures in the United States will triple to $45 billion by 2040 and more than double from there, to $102 billion by 2060.

† It is now believed that many components of the microbiome can be passed down through several generations and affect how our genes are expressed. In other words, great-grandchildren of Holocaust survivors or African Americans whose ancestors were slaves may still have physical manifestations of traumas suffered by people they never met.

microbiome is now seen as an integral part of our immune system that lives with us symbiotically. That understanding is revolutionizing the field of immunology* and offering new hope to patients suffering from autoimmune and inflammatory conditions. The concept of food as medicine has become accepted science. In many cases, it can reverse damaging inflammation.

Growing knowledge of how individual genomes interact with diet, drugs, circadian rhythms, and the microbiome can save millions of lives. Healthcare providers can more effectively treat malnutrition in children of developing nations because of their increased ability to correct microbiome imbalances.

EARLY DETECTION

Among other advances are the new types of mRNA vaccines to protect against COVID viruses. Alex Gorsky, then CEO of Johnson & Johnson, was one of my first podcast guests in April 2020. Even then, at the very early height of the crisis, he looked to the future with confidence:

> We have announced a lead vaccine candidate. This is a bit of a moonshot for us. Yet, history has shown major leaps forward after almost every crisis, whether it's a war, a natural disaster or a big challenge such as going to the moon. These force us to go in new directions, to collaborate and to accelerate technological breakthroughs.[†]

Eight months later, after the first vaccines had been approved, Alex returned for a second podcast. He was joined by Pfizer CEO

---

* Cell. 2014 Mar 27; 157(1): 121–141.

† https://mikemilken.com/podcast, episode 4; and later, episode 112.

Albert Bourla, who asked, "If we can develop these COVID vaccines in record time, why not new drugs for cancer, Alzheimer's, and other diseases?" I share that optimism and expect major advances in several areas. Among these are rapidly improving diagnostic tests that greatly improve the chances of curing diseases at their earliest stages. Cancer, for instance, was once considered an almost hopeless diagnosis. Now for some cancers, it's increasingly becoming a chronic disease we can live with. The overall death rate has already fallen by about 25 percent in just the last twenty years, largely because of progress on immunotherapy. For some cancers, survival times have doubled. In the future, scientists hope to develop vaccines that wipe out tumor cells before they even take shape. It's no exaggeration to say that the end of cancer as a cause of death and suffering is coming into sight.

The success of mRNA vaccines for COVID provides hope that personalized vaccines can now be developed fast enough to help cancer patients. These treatments have already shrunk tumors in mice.

The greatest recent gains have been in melanoma and liquid tumors. Solid tumors are the next challenge. Advanced cell therapy approaches more clearly define tumor components and then direct T cells to destroy them. Researchers are learning how to arrest tumor growth by throwing a "chemical switch" that disrupts cancer-causing genetic mutations.

Another interesting and potentially revolutionary perspective is to approach cancer as a computer science problem. David Soloveichik, PhD, a 1998 Milken Scholar, explains it this way:*

---

* Lori and I are very proud of what the more than 500 Milken Scholars have gone on to achieve. David Soloveichik was born in Kyiv, Ukraine, and brought to the United States by his parents as a child. He attended Harvard following his selection as one of our Scholars in 1998. David earned undergraduate and master's degrees in computer science at Harvard and then went to Caltech to study for his doctorate. His PhD dissertation on the mathematics of chemical reactions was awarded the Clauser Prize for the best doctoral thesis.

Killing cancer cells is easy. Doing it without killing healthy cells is hard. Eventually, we'll understand everything about how cancer cells communicate. At that point, curing cancer becomes an information processing process. We're still years away from that; but I'm completely confident we'll get there. Then we'll be able to make molecules do what we want them to do.

Perhaps the most exciting recent development in early detection is the multi-cancer blood test. A company called Grail now sells a simple test that it says accurately detects more than fifty types of cancer *across all stages* from a single blood draw.* The test has even found stage 1 localized cancer signals in such difficult diagnoses as pancreatic cancer. It achieves this by identifying tiny snippets of DNA that leak out of cancer cells into the bloodstream. At our 2021 Future of Health Summit, Grail's chief medical officer, Dr. Josh Ofman, described the state of cancer screening as analogous to an urban street with only a few streetlights scattered along one side. Most of the crime will occur on the unlit dark side of the street or in the dark gaps between the existing lights. Until recently, only five cancer types have had approved screening tests. The expansion to detection of fifty cancers could have a profound impact on public health by catching the 75 percent of malignancies "on the dark side of the street."

Other diagnostics companies, including Exact Sciences, are working toward similar tests. GuardantHealth of Germany claims 96 percent sensitivity in detecting early-stage colorectal cancer. These

---

He pursued further studies in synthetic biology at the University of Washington and at the University of California San Francisco. Dr. Soloveichik received the Feynman Prize in Nanotechnology from the Foresight Institute in 2012 and the Tulip Award from the International Society for Nanoscale Science, Computation and Engineering in 2014. He is now a professor at the University of Texas at Austin.

* In 2021, Illumina, Inc. announced its acquisition of Grail, but the transaction may be blocked by antitrust regulators. As this is written, the matter was unresolved.

kinds of screens are exciting because they have the potential to avert many deaths. The Milken Institute has joined more than thirty non-profit organizations in a Multi-Cancer Early Detection (MCED) consortium to evaluate such technologies.*

Multi-cancer screening is still at an early stage. As it improves, it may become a very powerful lifesaving resource. To illustrate its potential, best-selling author John Grisham wrote *The Tumor* (2016), a short fictional account of "Paul," a patient diagnosed with a fatal brain tumor. After nine months of ineffective treatments, Paul dies halfway through the book. The second part of the book retells the story ten years in the future. This time, Paul receives his diagnosis at a much earlier stage, when the tumor is small enough to be treated with focused ultrasound. Every few years, tumor cells reappear during routine checkups and the ultrasound treatment is repeated successfully.

John and I are fellow board members of the Focused Ultrasound Foundation and he is quick to acknowledge that his story is specu-lative. But he believes, as do I, in the great promise of these tech-nologies. In the not-too-distant future, getting a multi-cancer screen during a routine physical exam at your doctor's office may be as com-mon as getting your teeth x-rayed at the dentist's.

When cancer cells are first detected, before they appear on a radio-graphic scan, it will be easy to treat them with "smart bomb" drugs and possibly diet changes to energize and augment the immune sys-tem. If the cancer is more developed so that it appears as a small mass, your doctor may recommend a focused ultrasound treatment. Although *The Tumor* is a fictional story, confidence in such technol-ogies is sure to grow. They may become a great blessing for patients

---

* These tests have great potential, but can be expensive and are not without critics. Some worry about false positive results, patient costs, or pain from unnecessary treatments. To its credit, Grail has sponsored a large randomized trial to see how effective the tests are in actually reducing deaths.

who will no longer have to face difficult decisions about removal of a breast or a prostate.

Early detection also offers potential solutions for rare diseases. Thirty million Americans suffer from one of some six thousand of these conditions. Advances in knowledge of the human genome suggest we will be able not just to diagnose thousands of such devastating diseases at an early stage, but also to treat and even reverse them. We may soon be able to develop therapies for more than one disease at a time using sophisticated gene editing.

That's great news for parents of infants who suffer from rare, unexplained genetic conditions. They've often pursued a long, frustrating, and expensive search for answers when doctors can't figure out what's wrong with their sick babies. Now that widespread sequencing of newborns' genomes is practical, it's increasingly possible to diagnose and save more children.

AGING AND RESTORATION OF THE BODY

Widespread research on aging may one day lead to actual slowing of the aging process. Until then, various body restoration technologies are helping keep us functional and forestalling frailty in ways our grandparents couldn't imagine.

Surgery is becoming less dangerous and more effective. When focused ultrasound is not appropriate, an increasing proportion of surgeries can still avoid large incisions. Instead, surgeons treat patients with thin instruments and tiny cameras inserted through small ports.* With less damage to skin, muscles, and nerves, recovery

---

* Resistance to minimally invasive and robotic surgery by some surgeons was not surprising. New and improved technologies threaten people who are invested in the previous ways of doing things. Yet the success of the trend can be seen in the explosive market capitalization growth of leading companies in the industry. For example, the stock price of Intuitive

is faster with reduced pain. Another benefit: the bill is often lower because of shorter hospital stays.

Transplants of kidneys, hearts, livers, bones, coronary valves, skin, corneas, and other body parts have become increasingly common surgical procedures. Unfortunately, many patients die waiting because suitable tissue and organs are in short supply. Recent advances in experimental xenotransplantation from animals raises the prospect of more lifesaving procedures.

Kidneys may soon become widely available. Scientists are inbreeding pigs whose genes have been modified to eliminate the need for immunosuppression. For now, patients will still need harsh anti-rejection drugs, which carry risks of infection and cancer.

An even more advanced technique in the testing phase involves "educating" a patient's T cells not to attack the foreign cells of a transplant. Before transplantation of a kidney, for example, the patient receives an infusion of bone marrow from the donor. Antigens from the donor's marrow collect in the patient's thymus gland along with his own antigens. Later, the patient's T cells "respect" the donated kidney because they have seen its antigens in the thymus. The patient has become a chimera with two sets of antigens. This is still experimental, but potentially revolutionary.

Other scientists are engineering tissues to develop therapies and body parts produced from a patient's own cells. Some children born without a windpipe have received artificial tracheas built using their own stem cells over a matrix of plastic fibers. In 2022, a woman who had been born with an abnormal ear received a new ear that had been printed from her cells on a 3D printer.

For more than sixty years, people with sensorineural hearing loss have benefitted from cochlear implants, a neuroprosthesis that often

---

Surgical, which makes the Da Vinci Surgical System, increased by more than 700 percent from 2012 to 2022.

greatly improves understanding of speech. These devices have improved steadily and can transform a deaf or near-deaf person's quality of life. One study estimated that they can save up to $50,000 in special education costs when surgically implanted in a young child. Newer approaches to deafness include gene therapy, which is already bringing limited hearing to some deaf patients. Similarly, optogenetic therapy is restoring some vision to people blinded by retinal diseases. The improvements to date are marginal, but real, and are certain to continue.

The concept of organoids—multicellular *in vitro* tissue that mimics an *in vivo* human organ—is no longer science fiction. Researchers have created beating hearts and firing neurons in petri dishes. These miniature organs, sometimes called "mini me" tissue, suggest that we will eventually be able to grow functioning replacement organs, not just structural components like an ear or a trachea, from a patient's cells. In the foreseeable future, artificial kidneys, developed from what we know about stem cells and organoids, could free patients from the miserable experience of dialysis and save enormous healthcare resources.

Work has also begun on growing a type of artificial pancreas. It's a tremendous challenge, and success is far from assured, but someday it could cure juvenile diabetes. In the meantime, a "bionic pancreas" is already available. This automated mechanical device, which comes in various configurations, measures blood sugar and delivers insulin as needed to maintain reasonably good glycemic control.

LONGER LIVES

Not only are cures coming faster, but many of the remaining health threats, such as obesity, are within our control. Even the looming challenge of dementia has emerged as a major concern precisely because of our success against other diseases. Most people used to die from something else before encountering dementia. The following chart shows dramatic progress—despite the sharp impact of the 1918 flu pandemic and the recent setback from COVID-19.

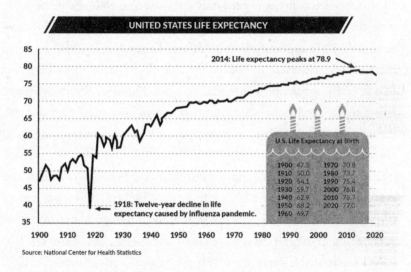

Source: National Center for Health Statistics

But here's an even more dramatic testament to the scientific method and public health:

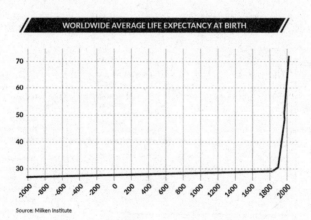

Source: Milken Institute

This chart is somewhat speculative. No one really knows exactly how long people lived in 1,000 BCE. With high infant and child mortality, the average life span was probably in the mid-to upper twenties. Those who made it to adulthood often reached their forties or beyond. Most demographic historians, however, agree that the hockey-stick shape is generally accurate and that the pivot point was the Industrial Revolution beginning around 1820. We do know that global life expectancy at birth was thirty-one in 1900 and had reached seventy-three by 2020. If you're lucky enough to be living in one of the wealthier countries, you can add several more years to the average. And remember that this shows life expectancy *at birth*. Those who retire healthy at seventy have a good chance of reaching their nineties.

Robert Fogel, the economic historian and Nobel laureate, was a popular panelist at the Milken Institute Global Conference before he passed away in 2013. The breadth of his interests was stunning—economics, demographics, physiology, the family, nutrition, the history of science, China's development, slavery, the American Civil War, and more. One year, he showed a chart with a line similar to the display of growing life expectancy on the previous page. What it

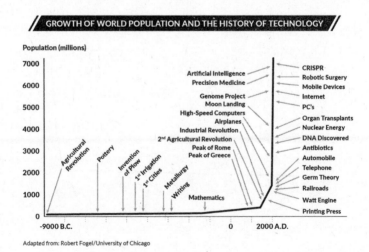

Adapted from: Robert Fogel/University of Chicago

shows, however, is not the length of life, but rather what those added years achieved by adding to the world's population and, more importantly, to our technology abundance.*

Bob Fogel's prediction of future life expectancy was optimistic: "It will probably increase the same amount during the twenty-first century as it did during the twentieth."

If you find it exciting to contemplate the idea of 110-year-old tennis players, consider this oft repeated statement from biomedical gerontologist Aubrey de Grey: "The first person to live to 150 is probably alive today." Bio-gerontology researchers say we're starting to understand the fundamental mechanisms of aging, which they believe is the first step to arresting and even reversing it. They hope that epigenetics will eventually allow us to switch off the cellular aging process.

Putting aside the predictions of futurists, I'm excited enough by the incredible progress we've already made and the acceleration of that progress by today's scientists. One of my favorite books on the subject is *Factfulness* by the late Swedish physician and global health advocate Hans Rosling. In a wonderfully iconoclastic way, Rosling celebrates what he calls "the secret silent miracle of human progress." He buttresses that with hundreds of optimistic facts such as this: Worldwide since 1800, the percent of children who die before age five has steadily declined from 44 percent to 4 percent. Over the same period, global literacy grew from one in ten to nine in ten.

TO THE FRONTIER

Back in 1995, my speech to the National Cancer Summit advocated "moving from a war of attrition to a plan of attack" and listed ten

---

* I've added some newer technologies that hadn't been developed in Fogel's lifetime.

road signs to follow. Today, we need greater concentration on ten areas at the frontiers of medical science:

1. Personalized mRNA vaccines to prevent most cancers and infections;

2. Noninvasive surgery;

3. Advanced nutrition to adjust the microbiome for optimal health;

4. CRISPR gene editing;

5. Multi-cancer screening;

6. Cell rejuvenation;

7. Advanced imaging for diagnosis and treatment of neurodegenerative diseases;

8. Immune system activation based on individualized genome sequencing;

9. Replacement organs grown from patients' own cells;

10. Implanted devices that provide twenty-four-hour measurement and responsive treatment.

One recent speaker at our Future of Health Summit was Eric Lefkofsky, the CEO of Tempus, a technology company that has built one of the world's largest libraries of clinical data and an operating system to make the data useful. A Tempus RNA sequencing test uses artificial intelligence to guide physicians about the diagnostic significance of a patient's tumor. Eric predicted that in fifty years, diseases like diabetes and cancer will seem as outdated as the idea of someone communicating by fax machine today. If that hardly seems possible, remember that the four-minute mile was once considered an impossible achievement. Yet soon after Roger Bannister broke through that psychological barrier in 1954, sixteen other runners beat the four-minute "limit" within a year. Science is about to beat many medical limits . . . to the great benefit of humanity.

*   *   *

REMAINING CHALLENGES AND YOUR CRUCIAL ROLE

President John F. Kennedy was touring the Cape Canaveral Space Center in 1962 when he spotted a man mopping the floor. At least that's how the story goes. JFK broke away from his entourage and greeted the fellow with a hearty "Hi! I'm Jack Kennedy. What are you working at?" Supposedly, the janitor replied, "Mr. President, I'm helping put a man on the moon." The thirty-fifth president liked to tell the story to emphasize the all-hands-on-deck requirements of the Apollo Program.

Our challenge of achieving cures for life-threatening diseases— faster cures—calls for the same breadth of commitment. It will take more than scientists. Each of us has a role. Every citizen, every patient, can be part of the solution. Here are a few things all of us can do:

- ◆ <u>Get involved.</u> Diseases don't care what political party you favor. Sensible public policies should be bipartisan, whether it's supporting funding for medical research or encouraging adherence to public health guidelines. Anyone can write a letter to the editor of a local newspaper, comment on a news website, or call the office of a legislative representative.

- ◆ <u>Get tested.</u> Lung cancer kills more Americans than any other form of cancer. Yet only about 15 percent of those most at risk have undergone the recommended CT scan. The numbers are better for colonoscopies, mammograms, Pap smears, and PSA tests—but still not as high as they should be. The result is that people are dying unnecessarily. Don't become one of those statistics.

+ Take personal responsibility for advancing health. If you're being treated for a medical condition, check out available clinical trials you might join. Places to ask include your doctor's office, a local hospital, or www.clinicaltrials.gov.

+ Avoid spreading misinformation on social media. If you know where to search, the internet can be a great source of information. Unfortunately, it's also full of quackery, misinformation and *dis*information. Before you pass along something you read, ask if it's from a reliable, objective source.

+ Advance science. Encourage bright students to pursue science careers. Buy a child a chemistry set or a telescope. Take kids to an aquarium, an observatory, or a science museum.

+ Observe public health guidelines. Keep up to date on all recommended vaccinations including an annual flu shot. If you have teenage children, make sure they've been immunized against the human papillomavirus. If you skipped the COVID-19 vaccinations, get them now.

+ Stay insured. Make sure your health insurance covers your needs and is up to date. Many studies have shown that insured patients live longer.

+ Collect, and give, your medical records. You have a right to receive copies of your health information. Always ask for them. Don't rely on your memory of old test results or the files of multiple doctors. The data could be very helpful years in the future when another provider assesses your medical history. It could also help researchers studying the prevalence of certain conditions or the impact of specific medications. Researchers are ethically and legally obligated to protect the privacy of your data, so be generous in authorizing its release.

+ Push back against inequities. A map of the New York City subway system tells something about health and the effect of where you live. As you travel north from midtown Manhattan to the South Bronx, life expectancy declines by ten years. That's six months for every minute on the train.*

Shocking statistics reported by Sir Michael Marmot, an epidemiologist at University College, London, make it clear that your zip code is more important than your genetic code when it comes to enjoying a long life.† Between the Chicago Loop and the west side of the city, the difference in life expectancy is sixteen years. In Baltimore's inner city, a man's life expectancy is sixty-three; not far away, in the Greater Roland Park/Poplar neighborhood, it's eighty-three. COVID helped to expose such disparities and stimulated efforts to address them.‡

*   *   *

If more of us take these actions, I believe they will have a real impact. As Margaret Mead once said, "Never doubt that a small group of thoughtful, committed citizens can change the world. Indeed, it's the only thing that ever has."

---

* Donald Berwick, MD, MPP "The Moral Determinants of Health," *Journal of the American Medical Association*, June 12, 2020.

† Michael Marmot, *The Health Gap*, Bloomsbury Press, 2015.

‡ The 2022 UP Summit in Bentonville, Arkansas, focused on the increased mobility people will enjoy using futuristic modes of transportation. My talk at the summit suggested that *social* mobility and equal access to healthcare were at least as important as physical mobility.

TWENTY-THREE

The Blessing of Meaningful Lives

More than four hundred years after Shakespeare wrote his plays and sonnets, they're as popular as ever. *Hamlet,* for example, is such an engrossing drama that movie studios and television networks produced seventy-one versions of this single play during the twentieth century. We recognize ourselves in the Bard's timeless themes because they deal with the basic human emotions that give our lives meaning.

SHAKESPEARE'S UNIVERSAL MESSAGES

NUMBER OF 20TH CENTURY FILM VERSIONS

Play	Key Messages	Films
Henry V	Honor, duty	8
King Lear	Pride, betrayal	14
Julius Caesar	Deceit, friendship	18
Romeo & Juliet	Love, fate, prejudice	37
Macbeth	Ambition, self-deception	39
Hamlet	Inner struggle, inaction	71

My pursuit of meaning followed the "three rivers" of my life described in this book's Introduction. In each, what gives my life meaning is a desire to help people, not only to create meaningful lives for themselves, but also to empower them to create meaningful lives for others. Elevating one teacher can elevate the thousands of students he or she will influence during a career; enabling gifted entrepreneurs to grow their businesses can create millions of jobs; supporting a medical researcher helps every patient worldwide who derives benefits from that physician-scientist's discoveries. As the poet Maya Angelou said in a 1990s Turner Broadcasting documentary about the American dream:

> *It may be, in fact, utterly impossible to be successful without helping another person to become successful . . . I don't think one can be liberated without liberating somebody else.*
>
> *[The American dream] is really no different than what is dreamed in Shanghai. It's the same dream that's dreamed in Cairo and Johannesburg. Everybody in the world wants a good job. Everybody in the world wants to be loved. Everybody wants healthy children. Everybody wants safe streets. Everybody wants to be able to count on good healthcare.*

That concept of a universal aspiration for the same goals motivated us to create the Milken Center for Advancing the American Dream (MCAAD). During the decade it has taken to create MCAAD, we recorded thousands of interviews with people in more than one hundred countries from every imaginable background. We always asked what the American dream meant to them. In many cases, they teared up as they told stories of a parent or grandparent whose sacrifices helped assure their success.

The MCAAD is an important part of our focus on meaningful lives. Whether a life has meaning should not be confused with living

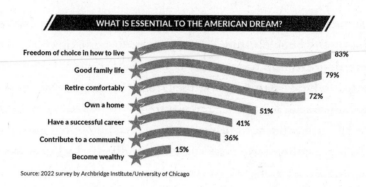

WHAT IS ESSENTIAL TO THE AMERICAN DREAM?

Freedom of choice in how to live — 83%
Good family life — 79%
Retire comfortably — 72%
Own a home — 51%
Have a successful career — 41%
Contribute to a community — 36%
Become wealthy — 15%

Source: 2022 survey by Archbridge Institute/University of Chicago

longer, earning credentials or accumulating assets. When the non-partisan Archbridge Institute conducts an annual survey about the essential components of the American dream, respondents consistently rank "Becoming Wealthy" as the least essential.

People feel their lives have been truly meaningful when they know they have made a positive difference to their families, their communities or their chosen field of work. We see the MCAAD as a beacon, a symbol of hope that no matter where you live, no matter your status in life, someday you will have a chance at your American dream.

AN EXTRAORDINARY THIRTY HOURS

I saw my own dream, the path I'd chosen in life, reflected in and affirmed by the hundreds of people I encountered in four cities—Boston, New York, Washington, and Los Angeles—beginning on Thursday afternoon, June 16, 2022, and ending late the next night. Collectively, these people represented the financial community, our medical research partnerships, and the Milken Institute centers in education, access to capital, public health, finance, and philanthropy.

After three weeks traveling the country, the twenty-sixth annual Home Run Challenge team was in the home stretch of visiting Major

League stadiums to raise cancer awareness and funds for research. As we walked out of Fenway Park, a man wearing a Boston Red Sox cap called my name. He wanted to shake my hand and thank me for a television interview I'd done a few years earlier urging men to talk to their doctors about a PSA test. As a result, he was diagnosed with prostate cancer at an early stage and had an excellent prognosis.

On my agenda later that evening was a New York event called Leveraged Finance Fights Melanoma (LFFM), which brought nine hundred financial professionals, melanoma patients and doctors together in the Sculpture Garden of the Museum of Modern Art. I was to cohost in the absence of Marc Hurlbert, CEO of the Melanoma Research Alliance (MRA), who'd been forced to quarantine after testing positive for COVID-19.

We arrived in time for me to greet several hundred attendees. Many were part of a cohort representing tens of thousands in the finance industry—private equity investors, issuers, money managers, rating evaluators, lawyers, analysts and others who have greatly expanded capital access. In the decades since the financial revolution of the 1970s, that industry has made the American dream more accessible to people everywhere by financing a far wider universe of entrepreneurs and job-creating businesses.

The driving force behind LFFM is Jeff Rowbottom, a senior financial executive and proud father of two daughters, who was diagnosed with melanoma in 2012. Surgery removed a large area of tissue on one of his legs. The cancer eventually returned, however, and he underwent more surgeries for lesions on his intestines. He then entered clinical trials for new immunology drugs—called PD-1 inhibitors—based on the work of Dr. James Allison. Today his cancer is in remission.

Jeff is now giving back by serving on the MRA board and devoting countless hours every year planning LFFM. That event has raised nearly $20 million for melanoma research.

Following that evening's formal program, Jeff and I joined three other attendees who have been closely involved in MRA programs. Each has a compelling story.

MOM'S FEARS

Ian Schuman is an experienced Wall Street lawyer who represents companies on high-profile securities offerings in the United States and around the world. Our discussion that night wasn't about finance, however. Instead, he began by telling me about his mother. In 2018, Ian explained to his parents that he had cancer throughout his body including his lungs, liver, spine and brain. "Seeing your mom cry in front of you—*about* you—is the ultimate worst experience." Until recent years, her assumption that her son was dying would have been correct—few survived cancer in the brain.

As a boy, Ian often played shirtless in the sun with no thought of applying sunscreen. Decades later, he discovered a lump near his collarbone. A biopsy identified melanoma and a PET scan showed widespread metastases. "At first, I felt extreme fear," said Ian. "Then, somehow, you find an extra gear and determine to punch back." Surgery alone was out of the question because the surgeon told him, "the cancer is everywhere." His oncologist, Dr. Jeffrey Weber, was blunt: "You have a massive cancer burden in your body."

Hope was not lost, however. The work of Jim Allison, whose research on immunology we began supporting in the mid-1990s, led to "checkpoint inhibitor" drugs, including Yervoy (ipilimumab). These compounds help release the immune system to fight cancer. Yervoy was approved by the FDA in 2011 for use in metastatic melanoma.

After three months of treatment with Yervoy in conjunction with

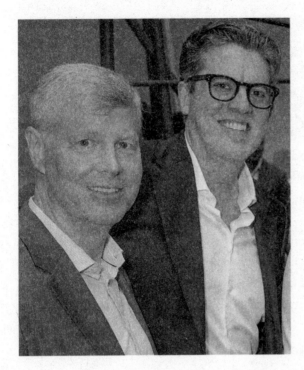

Ian Schuman (at right) joined Jeff Rowbottom at the June 16, 2022 fundraising event for melanoma research.

Opdivo, another immunotherapy drug, Ian had a follow-up scan. Looking at the radiology report, Dr. Weber said, "Congratulations, this is excellent." Three years later, Weber had even better news: "I'll follow you for ten more years, but there's no need for further treatment."

FORTY-TWO STAPLES

When Derrick Queen began to have severe headaches in 2016, he assumed they were caused by the stress of managing a hedge fund. But an MRI and other tests disclosed melanoma that had metastasized to three tumors in his brain, one larger than a golf ball. "After surgery, forty-two staples closed the incision across my forehead—

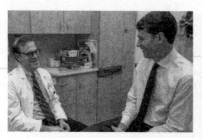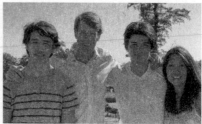

Left: Derrick Queen and oncologist Paul Chapman, MD; Right: Derrick with his wife, Vivian, and their sons Braden and Harrison.

it looked like the seams of a baseball." There was no way to hide the scar from his kids, then ages twelve and fourteen. He worried about how to tell them of his dire prognosis. What he can tell them now is that he's cancer-free thanks to immunotherapy and stereotactic radiation.

THERE FOR HIM

Lee Grinberg was engaged, but not yet married when, in 2013, a small lump on his shoulder turned out to be melanoma. His doctor sent him for a full body scan to check for any metastases. When the doctor's number popped up on his cell phone soon after the scan, Lee thought, *Uh-oh, this can't be good news.* There were two tumors in his brain. Within a few days, he was in surgery and then offered an experimental drug being developed with MRA support. His fiancée, Jenn, said she'd be there for him no matter what. Today they have three young children. Lee says that someday he will tell his kids they exist because of advanced treatments that were available to him.

I spoke to many patients and doctors that night. What struck

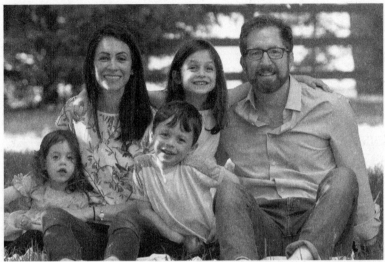

*Lee Grinberg with his wife, Jenn, and their children: Alexandra (top),
Eve, and Henry.*

me about Ian, Derrick, and Lee was that they'd all had cancer in
their brains—one of the last places you'd want to have cancer. Yet
here they were, healthy and thankful about their medical outcomes.
It was an emotional experience. After giving each of them a hug, I
couldn't help thinking that they were living examples of medical research progress. The major difference-maker is immunotherapy—a
true scientific miracle—that, unlike chemotherapy, doesn't kill
healthy cells. It takes the brakes off the immune system, which then
zeros in on the malignant cells.*

---

* Another grateful patient who had metastatic melanoma is former president Jimmy Carter. After being diagnosed with cancer in his liver and then his brain, he had surgery at the
age of ninety and was treated with the immunology drug Keytruda. Within months, his
scans showed him to be cancer-free. As this is written, President Carter is ninety-eight, our
nation's longest-lived president.

MORE STOPS ON THE TOUR

The Home Run Challenge tour, with a different city every day, was a grueling schedule. But arriving in Washington late that Thursday night after the LFFM event, I felt energized. The people I'd seen earlier that evening had reaffirmed our work in medical research and access to capital. The first of three scheduled meetings the next morning would center on education.

Our 7:00 a.m. breakfast session was a chance to congratulate the latest class of Scholars in the International Finance Corporation–Milken Institute Capital Markets Program at the George Washington University (GWU). These midcareer professionals from dozens of developing nations always inspire me with their optimism about the global economy's potential to overcome poverty and hunger. We spoke about the importance of creating meaningful jobs in their countries. I stressed that the American dream of social and economic mobility is for people everywhere.

Breakfast number two was for the Prostate Cancer Foundation. Mark Ein, a successful entrepreneur and philanthropist I've known for decades, served as host and introduced my talk about twenty-six years of research progress supported by the Home Run Challenge. Also joining us were several other longtime friends including Ed Cohen, a principal owner of the Washington Nationals baseball team, and Dr. Kurt Newman, CEO of Children's National Hospital.

Frank Luntz, the TV commentator, communications consultant and university professor, hosted the morning's third meeting. Frank, who teaches a college course for NYU Abu Dhabi students from around the world, asked me to speak to these young scholars and answer their questions. They represented countries as industrially advanced as Japan and as desperately poor as South Sudan. Their course in Washington allowed them to study the US political system from all sides of the partisan spectrum and to meet with journalists, members of Congress and other policy leaders. One young Sudanese man shared his personal experience of having to flee with his family from his home, which was surrounded by teenage guerrilla soldiers toting assault rifles, to the "safety" of a refugee camp in Ethiopia. He said he would never take freedom for granted.

Now it was time for the day's Home Run Challenge game at Nationals Park, where we hosted about fifty guests. (The Philadelphia Phillies edged the Nats 5–3 and I spoke to broadcast viewers about the goals and achievements of medical research.)

MILES TO GO

The second part of the day was just getting started. A quick ride across town brought me to the Constitution Avenue headquarters of the United States Federal Reserve, our nation's central bank. At the time, economic pundits were debating whether the Fed could successfully engineer a "soft landing" by raising interest rates to reduce inflation while not causing a severe recession. I exchanged ideas with Fed Chairman Jay Powell based on our work at the Milken Institute. Then I mentioned the famous foreign policy dictum of Teddy Roosevelt: "Speak softly and carry a big stick." To the chairman's surprise, my advice was to do just the opposite: "Speak loudly and carry a small stick." My point was that when someone in his position talks loudly about some potential action, people respond by adjusting their behavior. In this case, the "smaller stick" of less-drastic interest rate increases might be all that's needed. It's not clear whether he agreed, but a few days later he told Congress, loudly, (or as loudly as is possible in Fed-speak), "We think [higher interest rates] are absolutely essential to bring down inflation." In response, a significant source of inflation—commodity markets prices—promptly fell.

Next on the day's agenda was a reception at the Milken Center for Advancing the American Dream, then in preparations for its 2024 public opening. We greeted a group of Washington, DC, leaders and spoke about some of the Center's exciting plans built around its four pillars: education and the educator; public health and medical research; access to capital and financial empowerment; and entrepreneurship and innovation.

SUMMING UP THE BLESSINGS

That evening, as our plane took off to the west and the Virginia countryside fell away from view, anticipation of a five-hour flight put me in a contemplative mood. Starting in Boston, then New York, and now heading from Washington to Los Angeles, my journey felt like far more than a quick four-city trip. I had experienced the missions of my adult life summarized in little more than twenty-four hours.

As we flew across the Midwest, the late-June sun finally set and my mind wandered across decades—the 1960s, when a man on a riot-torn street in Watts awakened my sense of social disparities and inspired my theories of access to capital; the 1970s, when we played a key role in the success of a new financial system and put increased focus on support of medical research on pediatric neurology; the 1980s, when we launched our education initiatives and expanded medical programs; the 1990s, when we built on previous philanthropy to change the infrastructure and processes of education and medical research; the early 2000s and the maturing of a strategy for bioscientific innovation; the 2010s that included expansion of our public health initiatives; and the current decade's mobilization to confront COVID and prepare for a future of greatly improved health worldwide.

Crossing the Continental Divide, and heading southwest toward home, I thought of the links from past events with my personal interactions since the previous evening in New York—our increased support of immunotherapy research and Jim Allison's 1997 statement that the immune system is smarter than all of us. Without Jim's Nobel Prize–winning work, the melanoma survivors I was able to hug the night before surely would not have made it. Gary Becker's insights about human capital beginning in the 1960s had informed so many of our programs in education and economic development around the world. The many entrepreneurs whose growing businesses I'd financed in the 1970s and '80s now paid it forward by becoming substantial philanthropists supporting programs in public health and medical research.

Lori was waiting when I arrived home before midnight. It was almost Saturday. Our last two Home Run Challenge contests were Dodgers home games, just a few miles away. Sunday's game was on Father's Day and we planned a multi-generational family outing at the stadium.

The gift of time with family and close friends since my cancer diagnosis has been an incredible treasure. Nothing matches the blessing of more than sixty years with Lori and seeing our children grow up, get married, and have kids of their own. My last thought before falling asleep with her was how very fortunate I am.

Acknowledgments

My gratitude to the thousands who have worked with me for half a century to produce improved health outcomes—physicians, scientists, academic medical leaders, biopharmaceutical executives, and government health officials, plus the patients who volunteer for clinical trials—is unbounded. Their insights and accomplishments have changed the world. If not for them, I wouldn't be here.

Special thanks to Andy von Eschenbach, caring physician and good friend, for writing this book's foreword. Also . . . Geoffrey Evans Moore, my coauthor, who has been a steadfast partner and adviser for a quarter century . . . Mauro DiPreta, Andrew Yackira, and the others on the HarperCollins team who made many perceptive suggestions . . . Andrew Stuart, our agent, whose counsel helped the project take shape . . . My wife Lori, whose editorial observations were invaluable . . . and Genie Gable, whose comments on successive drafts improved the narrative.

Heartfelt appreciation for the accomplishments of hundreds of colleagues at the Milken Institute, the Milken Family Foundation, the Prostate Cancer Foundation, *FasterCures*, the Milken Institute

School of Public Health, the Milken Center for Advancing the American Dream, the Center for Strategic Philanthropy, the Center for the Future of Aging, the Center for Public Health, the Center for Financial Markets, the Melanoma Research Alliance, and Knowledge Universe. They have built our programs over the decades and given me deeper perspectives on the topics addressed in this book.

Encouragement from my extended four-generation family, and especially from Lori, has given me strength and courage in our continuing search for faster cures.

Photo Credits

Images in the text are courtesy of the author, except:

p. 11, courtesy *Pictorial Parade* via Getty Images; p. 21, courtesy New York Daily News Archive via Getty Images; p. 37, courtesy Bettmann via Getty Images; p. 41, courtesy the Los Angeles Times, © 2015; p. 44, courtesy © 1962 by the University of Chicago. All rights reserved. Gary S. Becker, "Irrational Behavior and Economic Theory." *The Journal of Political Economy* 70, no. 1 (1962): 1–13. Published by the University of Chicago Press; p. 46, courtesy Princeton University Press. *Corporate Bond Quality and Investor Experience* by W. Braddock Hickman, published 1968; p. 85, courtesy Bettmann via Getty Images; p. 105, courtesy Steven Rubin; p. 116, (left) courtesy Chicago Booth Marketing, (right) courtesy Dan Dry, courtesy of *The University of Chicago Magazine*; p. 302, courtesy Clark S. Judge; p. 325, courtesy Melanoma Research Alliance; p. 326, (left) courtesy Lara Porzak, (right) courtesy Derrick Queen; p. 327, courtesy Lee Grinberg

Images in the photo insert are courtesy of the author, except:

p. 1, (center) by Brodie Port; p. 2, (top left) courtesy of Providence Saint John's Cancer Institute; (top middle) courtesy of National Cancer Institute; (top right) courtesy of the Reginald F. Lewis Foundation; p. 3, (top, second from left) courtesy of National Cancer Institute/Linda Bartlett; (second from bottom) courtesy of Weill Cornell Medicine; p. 5, (top left) courtesy of *Newsweek* magazine, December 16, 1985 edition, (top right) courtesy of National Institutes of Health, (center left) courtesy of Children's National Hospital, (bottom) from *Forbes*, December 15, 2014, © Forbes. All rights reserved. Used under license; p. 6, (bottom) used with permission of Bloomberg Businessweek, copyright © 2022. All rights reserved; p. 7, (top left) courtesy of Institute for Systems Biology, (top right) by Christopher Michel; p. 13, (top) White House photo by Pete Souza, (bottom left and bottom right) courtesy of Milken Institute SPH; p. 15, (top left) courtesy of AP Photo/Patrick Semansky. Photos by Paul Bliese: p. 4, center and bottom; p. 5, center middle and center right; p. 6, top; p. 7, center; p. 8, bottom; p. 9, top and bottom; p. 10, top left, top right, center left, and center right; p. 11, all; p. 12, all; p. 13, center; p. 15, top right; p. 16, bottom

Index

About the Authors

———————

Michael Milken's career has mirrored his four main professional passions: medical research, education, public health, and access to capital. He has been uniquely successful in creating value, whether measured in lives saved (*Fortune* magazine called him "The Man Who Changed Medicine"), students inspired (*Forbes* said he is an education visionary), or jobs created. Beginning in 1969, he financed thousands of companies that collectively created millions of jobs. Members of the team that worked with him lead many of today's major financial institutions, and Milken's innovations are the basis for much of modern capital markets structure.

His philanthropy, which began in the 1970s and paralleled his business career, expanded in 1982 with the establishment of the Milken Family Foundation. After two decades of actively supporting medical research, he became a patient in 1993 when he was diagnosed with terminal cancer. Over the last three decades, he has increased his focus on making the research process more effective and efficient.

Milken also chairs the Milken Institute, a widely respected think tank whose annual Global Conference brings more than four thousand leaders from fifty nations to Los Angeles. Other annual conferences are held in London, Washington, DC, Singapore, and the Middle East. The Milken Institute School of Public Health at George Washington University was renamed in recognition of a gift from the Institute.

He graduated from Berkeley with highest honors and earned his MBA at the Wharton School, where he was a Joseph Wharton fellow. He and his wife, Lori, who are members of the Giving Pledge, have been married since 1968. They have three children and ten grandchildren.

Geoffrey Evans Moore is a communications consultant and a Milken Institute senior advisor. Moore has written frequently about public policy issues in major publications. He was previously a senior vice president at Dow Jones and served for twenty-two years in communications management and executive speechwriting positions for IBM in the US and Japan. Earlier, he was an assistant to New York governor Nelson Rockefeller, press secretary to US Senate Minority Leader Hugh Scott, and Director of Public Information for the US Equal Employment Opportunity Commission. He is a graduate of the University of Pennsylvania.